Health Issues for Women of Color

N

O

N

D

This book is dedicated to my daughter, Dawn; my niece, Patricia; and to six very special young girls—Alea, Alycia, Danyelle, Kaebah, Teale, and Zaida, as well as all young girls of color.

Health Issues for Women of Color

A Cultural Diversity Perspective

Diane L. Adams, M.D., editor

SAGE Publications
International Educational and Professional Publisher
Thousand Oaks   London   New Delhi

For information address:

SAGE Publications, Inc.
2455 Teller Road
Thousand Oaks, California 91320
E-mail: order@sagepub.com

SAGE Publications Ltd.
6 Bonhill Street
London EC2A 4PU
United Kingdom

SAGE Publications India Pvt. Ltd.
M-32 Market
Greater Kailash I
New Delhi 110 048 India

Printed in the United States of America

Library of Congress Cataloging-in-Publication Data

Main entry under title:

Health issues for women of color : a cultural diversity perspective /
    edited by Diane L. Adams.
        p. cm.
    Includes bibliographical references and indexes.
    ISBN 0-8039-7311-X — ISBN 0-8039-7312-8 (pbk.)
    1. Minority women—Health and hygiene—United States. 2. Minority
women—Medical care—United States. 3. Minority women—United
States—Social conditions. 4. Homeless women—Health and hygiene—
United States. 5. Homeless women—Medical care—United States.
6. Homeless women—United States—Social conditions. I. Adams,
Diane L. (Diane Loretta).
RA564.86.H43 1995
362.1′08′693—dc20   95-4400

    96 97 98 99 10 9 8 7 6 5 4 3 2

This book is printed on acid-free paper.

Cover design: Adrian Wong Shue.

Disclaimer: The views expressed by the various authors in this publication do not represent the views of agencies or institutions with whom they are affiliated.

Contents

Foreword

I am honored to have been asked by Diane Adams to write the foreword for this book. This is a book by women about women. It provides a broad, comprehensive perspective on both the strengths and challenges related to women's health. The strengths emerge in the many different roles that women have played throughout history, resulting in major contributions to the health and well-being of communities and society. Women have many responsibilities: They are educators, students, comforters, nurturers, mothers, elders, leaders, peacekeepers, healers, and homemakers.

Many positive, culturally relevant, constructive efforts throughout the United States today are likely to affect women's wellness. This text addresses contemporary women's health outcomes and examines the impact of cultures on women's health. The underlying theme of this text is that women of all colors and ethnic groups can achieve a higher level of health and wellness.

Sometimes people pick up books devoted to women and assume that the underlying message is about hating or disliking men. That is not the premise of this book, although it has little to do *directly* with men. Instead, it is an opportunity to examine women of all colors.

This book is a journey into women's health, well-being, strengths, and growth.

But as the book unfolds, readers will also see the many tragedies that continue to confront women. The traumas and problems that women confront today, such as sexual abuse, domestic violence, drug abuse, cultural/sexual stereotyping, racism and discrimination, HIV infection, and homelessness, are described in some depth. The purpose of these descriptions is to provide a comprehensive base upon which women-specific health problems and disorder prevention programs may be founded.

Among the many challenges that professionals face when initially working in women's health is the dearth of accurate data to support the development of culturally competent women's health programs. The descriptive summaries of women's traumatic circumstances provide an overview of the many health problems common among women in today's society. It is easy to become upset when reading about the plight of women of all colors who are homeless, or victims of abuse, or incarcerated. It is difficult to read of women who have been brutally beaten or humiliated. It is easy to feel rage. It is harder to do something constructive about that anger. I strongly encourage readers to select the harder choice and to move beyond rage. Take the data and descriptions presented in this book and *do* something constructive with that new knowledge or perception. For a busy professional, homemaker, or student, this may mean volunteering one evening a month at a homeless shelter or assisting with an educational program for incarcerated women. It may mean giving up one's own anger and rage over undeserved trauma and abuse and helping others work through their own resentment. Or it can mean becoming a major contributor, like Dr. Vivian Pinn (Director of the Office of Research on Women's Health of the National Institutes of Health), who is responsible for national women's initiatives providing opportunity for more women to be in leadership roles on women's research projects.

As described within this text, the current health status of women of color is significantly inferior to that of middle-class white women. The leading causes of death within each ethnic and racial group have some similarities (e.g., cardiovascular disease) and yet are different in many ways. It is generally not known whether the variations of morbidity and mortality among races and cultures are due to culture, environment, or genetic predisposition. As data are collected on women of color, patterns evolve that show differences between men and women of the same ethnic and racial group. The factors that influence these differences are largely unknown. For example, data indicate that African American males do *not* respond as well as white males when treated with the same medication for a specific type of cancer. Variations of physical response to medication may also be *gender*-specific.

As with all underserved populations, poverty and education play major roles in misconceptions about women of color. All too often, contemporary media carry news only about the disturbances, not the triumphs, of women of color. The public perception is frequently biased, showing African American or Hispanic women on welfare to the exclusion of their paler sisters.

With more and more women attaining academic degrees and professional skills, there is great opportunity to develop and implement culturally competent social and health programs for and by women. It is hoped that within the near future, enough high-quality data will be available so that the disproportionate health problems of women of color are no longer highlighted, but rather the demonstrated effectiveness of programs developed by and for women of color.

Issues of racism and discrimination are incorporated in several chapters. Young students frequently express surprise that such attitudes continue to flourish in this country and occasionally challenge claims that racism exists. Racism has been exemplified in many ways in contemporary society, and it is evident even during pleasurable leisure activities, like crowds performing the "tomahawk chop" during baseball games. Likewise, many laws that reinforce racism are still on the books. For example, as of 1995, Missouri law states that anyone who claims to be an Indian can be shot or hung on sight.

As a result of racism, readers are likely to encounter women of color who are in the process of discovering the richness and beauty of their individual cultures. This process of accepting themselves sometimes contributes to the racial misclassification in federal, state, and local databases. For example, some women self-report themselves as one race one day and a year later identify themselves as belonging to another race. This is not uncommon and usually occurs while a woman is learning to be comfortable with herself, her culture, and her potential. This shifting of cultural identity reflects the challenges inherent in becoming an empowered and self-confident woman who appreciates who and what she is.

However, cultural identity also carries with it a responsibility. For example, Bennett (1992) describes self-identity as an Indian as follows:

> Being Indian is more than checking the box for ethnic origin. It is a way of life, a way of being. The love for family, respect for your elders, spirituality, self-determination, integrity, pride, understanding, protecting the environment, humor, and socializing are all the essence of being Indian.

Similar perceptions and responsibilities exist for other cultures.

Many opportunities exist for women to meet together and discuss strategies for improving the plight of women and women of color. It is interesting to note how often women refer to the cultural strengths and powers that women possessed within their own cultures in recent history. For example, a common theme or concept is "becoming healthy again." This concept refers to the many healthy lifestyles that were practiced by one's ancestors and that help prevent disease and promote health.

Among the themes which infiltrate each author's chapters and perspectives on women's health issues is the need to acknowledge and respect the woman's ethnic culture, and simultaneously to respond to the diversity that is apparent in each group of women and within each group of women of color. Most underserved cultures have strong social structures. The family frequently is the focal point of most activities and practices. The woman's role within that family unit varies tremendously within the social structure of each culture. These diverse roles are clarified in several of the early chapters of the text.

While reviewing the chapters, the reader needs to also acknowledge the commonalities that exist among almost all women, for example, the well-being of one's family. When women get together and talk about the challenges of raising children, coping with work and managing a home, dealing with a partner who sits for hours on end before the television watching sports events, and/or creating and maintaining a productive relationship with a friend or partner, women of all ethnic groups usually find at least one of these to be "common ground" on which to base a relationship. It really doesn't matter whether the women are Norwegian, Kenyan, Native Hawaiian, Vietnamese, or Choctaw. These specific ethnic identities and cultural distinctiveness shadow in the midst of these commonalities.

However, the *ways* one adapts to these common events, such as raising our children, is greatly affected by culture. For example, during an intertribal gathering, young toddlers were running around and playing near an open fire pit. As the children moved closer to the fire, an Indian mother also moved closer, but made no attempt to prevent the children from playing in the area. A non-Native woman who was present began to express her concern about the children being unsupervised. The Indian mother was rather insulted and responded that she was supervising the children. During the subsequent discussion, the non-Native woman expressed her feelings about the need to prevent the children from playing in an area where they were exposed to danger, such as fire. The Indian woman responded that if a child were to get too close, she would allow the child to get near the fire, but not to be injured, and the value of this "lesson" was that the child would always be careful and respectful of fire in the future. Both women love and care for their children, but their cultural philosophies of raising the child regarding safety behaviors was quite extreme from one another.

Women are confronted with many erroneous stereotypes. Several of the chapters combat those stereotypes by presenting empirical data and/or descriptions which leaves the reader questioning how such silly stereotypes ever emerged. For example, in the Zambrana and Ellis chapter, the reader is introduced to the cultural diversity which exists among Hispanic and Latina women. Meleis and Hattar-Pollara elaborate on the blatant and subtle manners in which Arab Middle Eastern American Women are stereotyped. Tom-Orme provides an overview of the severity of health problems confronting Indian women today that presents a different picture from those displayed in most media. Eng describes women of domestic violence in a manner which helps the reader realize that these people frequently do not "fit" the stereotype presented in news stories and novels.

Among the unique features of this text is the emphasis on homeless women and their families. Chapters 11, 12, 13, and 14 describe mental health problems, the process of coping with raising children while homeless, the difficulty of getting access to health care, and prospective trends likely to emerge in our societies regarding homeless women and their children. The chapters effectively eradicate stereotypes and clarify that homelessness is much more than an issue or effect of poverty alone. The many ramifications of homelessness on women within their country as well as its subsequent effects on U.S. society cannot continue to be ignored.

This publication is of acceptance and appreciation of diversity and its subsequent effects of women's health. It is a journey through empowerment that is at times frustrating and at other times exhilarating. Although every human being is blessed with many special gifts and skills, there is a need to continue to develop and implement culturally relevant and competent health programs within our communities. This publication isn't just about gaining a comprehensive perspective . . . it is about taking that perspective and making a constructive contribution to preventing women's health problems and promoting women's health and wellness. I encourage you, the reader, to enjoy the diversity that is represented in this publication and to use the new knowledge and understanding of these many different facets, issues, and challenges of women's health to make a contribution of your own.

LINDA BURHANSSTIPANOV
Director, Native American
Cancer Research Program

Reference

Bennett, S. K. (1992). The American Indian: A psychological overview. In *Psychology of culture* (pp. 35-39). Needham Heights, MA: Allyn & Bacon.

Acknowledgments

Special Acknowledgment

To Dr. Raymond L. Blakely, Chairman of the Department of Physical Therapy, and to my aunt and uncle, Dr. Dennis and Mrs. Fannie Perry, who have believed in me and provided an atmosphere for growth.

Mentors

To C. Alex Alexander, MD, Veterans Administration Medical Center; Christopher G. Chute, MD, Mayo Clinic; Gertrude T. Hunter, MD, Human Services Education and Research Institute, Inc.; Carroll M. Leevy, MD, New Jersey Medical School; Audrey F. Manley, MD, Acting Surgeon General and Deputy Surgeon General—U.S. Public Health Service; Edith H. Schoenrich, MD, Johns Hopkins University School of Hygiene and Public Health; Robert Veiga, MD, U.S. Public Health Service; and Henry W. Williams, MD, Howard University Hospital—Department of Community Health and Family Practice, who provided support in all my endeavors.

Honorable Mention

Honorable mention is gratefully extended to the following individuals who were instrumental in various ways in making this book a reality and/or giving undying support to my many other efforts. These people have believed in my dream and have in both big and little ways encouraged me. Bernice S. Reyes-Akinbileje, Diana Axelsen, Deby Blum, L. Robert Bolling, Dr. America Bracho, Darrell Brown, Dr. Lucile Adams-Campbell, Senator Ben Nighthorse Campbell (Colorado), Dora Carrington, Elizabeth M. Carson, Dr. Amy Cato, Barbara Clark, Shirley Clark, Violet P. Cherry, Congresswoman Cardiss Collins (Illinois), Felicia L. Collins, Mimi Conner, Michael Coulter, Dr. Jane Delgado, Diana Dodd, Dr. Wynne DuBray, Dr. Edward V. Ellis, Harriett Epps, Dr. Eric Farag, Dr. Rosalyn P. Epps, Nancy Williams Fisher, Dr. Bridgie Alexis Ford, Cherrie Foster, Romona S. Fullman, Tessie Guillermo, Dr. Freda Lewis-Hall, Kristy Heflin, Dr. Portia Hunt, Dr. William P. Hytche, Dr. Jennie R. Joe, Delores W. Johnson, Eva Johnson, Michone Trinae Johnson, Kim Canavan Jones, Thurman D. Jones, Jr., Dr. Kunle Kassim, Mapolean King, Siani Lee, Sharon Lillie, Ginger Lindbergh, Olivier Denier Long, Clotine Mason, Margaret S. Mason, Floydetta McAfee, Dr. Lorna S. McBarnette, Dr. Beatrice Medicine, Gertrude T. McClairen, Renee McCullough, Dan Mroczkowski, Stanley J. Phillips, Gig and Howard Pimpleton, Dr. Vivian Pinn, Dr. Francis Plummer, Dr. Marion E. Primas, Dr. John Robinson, Dr. LaFrancis Rodgers-Rose, Dr. Edgar E. Roulhac, Charlene Russell, Gayle Sexton, Shawnn K. Shears, Martha Sherman, Adrian Wong Shue, Sue Simon, Christine Smedley, Cheryl A. Smith, Ellevia L. Smith, Congressman Louis Stokes (Ohio) and staff (Leslie Atkinson, Joyce Larkin, Neal O'Hara, Joanne White), Fannie Thompson, Dr. H. R. Treadwell, Dr. C. Delores Tucker, Faith Wall, Jeanette J. Washington, Sallie E. Welch, Jean Wicks, Dr. Donald E. Wilson, to all contributing writers, all the participants from the 16 states, District of Columbia, and Canada, who attended the First National Conference on Cultural Diversity and Women's Health, Women of Color: A Major Challenge for Health Care Reform, held June 12-13, 1993, at the Lord Baltimore Hotel (Radisson), Baltimore, Maryland, and all of the participants in the soiree, jointly sponsored by the Office of Women's Health, Maryland Department of Health and Mental Hygiene, and the Cultural Diversity and Women's Health Program, University of Maryland Eastern Shore at the Region III Official Preparatory Conference for the Fourth World Conference on Women (held in Wilmington, Delaware, on August 4, 1994, by the U.S. Department of Labor, Women's Bureau) to be held in Beijing, People's Republic of China, Summer of 1995.

The June 1993 conference would not have been possible without the generous grant from the Kellogg Foundation and Marion Merrill Dow, Inc.

And last, but by no means least, to former Governer William Donald Schaefer of Maryland, who while in office issued a proclamation in support of the initial effort to establish a Cultural Diversity and Women's Health Program at the University of Maryland Eastern Shore.

Family

To Kareem and Akeem, who provided the support that only two sons can give.

To Bill, my husband, who has shared my dreams and even encouraged me to dream.

1 Introduction

DIANE L. ADAMS

BETTY SMITH WILLIAMS

Effective health care in the United States demands that attention be given to all people. Historically, it has been found that the specific health problems of women have been given less serious attention in the areas of research and treatment than the problems of men. Only recently, after pressure was applied, Congress required inclusion of women in federally funded health research. The result of the years of neglect has been a serious deficit in knowledge about health problems specific to women. This deficit is compounded for health problems distinctive to women of color and their subgroups. Such lack of information greatly diminishes the competency of health providers to identify health problems and their related behaviors and therefore impairs their ability to deliver effective care to women of color.

It is generally recognized that traditional health care delivery has failed in its mission of providing health outcomes of equal quality to women of color and diverse cultures, a growing segment of the population that needs culturally competent care by health professionals. The challenge before us is to create effective health policy and health delivery that accommodate the racial, economic, cultural, and ethical issues affecting health care delivery to distinct groups and subgroups of women of color.

This book presents a multidisciplinary and multifaceted approach to the health care concerns of women of color, within the context of the impact cultural diversity has upon health care. The authors' presentations acknowledge and recognize the major classifications of women of color and their subgroups, as well as the distinct challenges of serving them.

In assembling the contents, the intent was to provide a volume useful to graduate educators of various disciplines, professionals in private practice, those providing primary as well as personal health care, researchers, and policymakers, as well as lay people—mothers, sisters, aunts, uncles, fathers, brothers, husbands, and wives. The book should also be of value to high school and undergraduate school educators and students, and to any and everyone in any way affected by women's health.

The health of women is viewed through their various roles as caregivers, wives, mothers, and family stabilizers/heads of households. Among the topics included are domestic violence, anxiety, drug abuse, mental health, homelessness, sexism, and racism. Within some cultural groups, such topics are taboo and/or seldom explored outside the confines of their particular group.

Besides identifying the prevailing health problems and their historical prevalence in each of the major groups of women of color, the book also examines health promotions/wellness paradigms and health prevention, as well as intervention strategies.

Readers are made aware of related health concerns and the emotional, social, economic, ethical, and environmental issues that have an impact on the health—both physical and mental—of women of color, who have vastly diverse heritages from subgroup to subgroup and even within subgroup. The multidimensional view enlightens readers about the extent of what must be done to bring parity to health care for women of color. It also provides insight into the importance of cultural sensitivity and cultural competence in eliminating barriers to access to health care.

It is fitting that the initial discussions of the book are about the health of the first U.S. women, American Indian/Alaskan Natives. Hispanic/Latina women and Asian/Pacific Islander women are subjects of following chapters, each group with apparent high growth potential in the United States. African American women, a long-standing population in this country, have unique issues and share circumstances applicable across the diverse cultures of women of color. Subsequent chapters address emerging health concerns and the future of research. The final chapter focuses on women of color from a population newer to the United States, women of Middle Eastern cultures.

Several authors identify the key health policy implications drawn from their analysis of the status of particular cultural groups. The importance of accurate data collection about diverse subgroups within cultures is emphasized. If it is not considered, the great variability within cultural groups can mean professionals use misleading data and overlook serious health problems. The implications for research design, methodology, and interpretation are substantial.

The strengths of women of color and diverse cultures are emphasized throughout the discussions. Authors focus upon specific strengths and solutions that should guide providers and policymakers. Identifying strengths upon which to build interventions is of great importance. Many discussions of people of diverse cultures assess the deficits and emphasize the differences. This new data approach promises to help find new interventions that meet the challenge to provide excellent, culturally competent care for women of color.

The book's contributors are a diverse group of women of color who are health care professionals from various disciplines and cultures. Internationally recognized authorities bring state of the art knowledge from their learned and cultural perspectives to enrich readers.

It is anticipated that the information provided in this book will create an awareness of the many needs that must be met in specific areas to bring about a significant and recognizable improvement in the health care of women of color. For example, this book should encourage the inclusion of women's health issues/problems in the curriculum of study in medical education. Attention should be given to developing courses designed to create positive attitudes toward the treatment of women's health problems in general and the health problems characteristic of women of color in particular. Such courses should emphasize the importance and necessity of incorporating and using cultural strengths of specific groups to arrive at desired health outcomes. Some attention needs to be given to the significance of cultural diversity and the need for cultural sensitivity and cultural competence in the education curriculum of all health care providers. All health professional associations need to develop continuing education programs in women's health and cultural diversity.

Representative samples of women of color must be included in research studies, particularly those that focus on health problems that result in significantly disproportionate and high morbidity and mortality rates among women of color. Also needed are research studies that focus on improving health outcomes in specific health conditions peculiar to women of color.

Finally, this book aims to shed light on the need for and the challenge to develop effective public policy regarding women of color and cultural diversity—policy that considers racism, economics, culture, and ethnic and ethical practices.

2 Cultural Diversity and Institutional Inequality

AIDA L. GIACHELLO

In recent years there has been an increased interest in addressing the health needs of culturally diverse populations in the United States. However, the needs of women of color have been consistently ignored in many of the health policy discussions. This chapter is aimed at providing some basic definitions of terms that will be used throughout this book. These are terms that we often hear or use without a clear understanding of their meanings. The terms that will be defined are *culture, race* and *racial groups, ethnicity* and *ethnic groups, minorities, prejudice, social discrimination, cultural knowledge, cultural awareness, cultural competence, the melting pot ideology, affirmative action, quota system,* and *cultural diversity.* This chapter will then provide some explanations about the current interest in cultural diversity issues and some of the barriers that must be overcome to properly address the needs of women of color. Finally, this chapter will suggest policy recommendations, accompanied by specific strategies to achieve institutional equality.

Some Basic Terms

Culture. Culture is a dynamic pattern of learned behaviors, values, and beliefs exhibited by a group that shares history and geographic proximity. It refers to everything we learn in the process of socialization. Children and adolescents are socialized to assume gender-defined roles and obligations that place women in a socially disadvantaged position in reference to men. With respect to health and illness, the culture socializes the individual as to how to think, act, and feel toward illness. It determines the health attitudes and behaviors and the roles of the actors—the healer (the physician) and the patient.

Race and Racial Groups. Racial group and the common term race have been used in a number of ways in social sciences and in popular writings. The earliest use of race in 16th- and 17th-century Europe was in the sense of descendants of a common ancestor, emphasizing kinship linkages (Feagin, 1989). Since the 18th century, race has been given a biological and social meaning. It means a distinct category of human beings with physical characteristics transmitted by descent (Feagin, 1989, p. 5). From the social perspective, the term racial groups refers to groups that define themselves and/or are defined by others as different by virtue of (presumed) innate and immutable physical characteristics (Feagin, 1989). Certain physical characteristics, such as skin color, are selected as a basis for distinguishing the members of the group.

Ethnicity and Ethnic Groups. Ethnic groups are those that can be distinguished by socially selected cultural characteristics, such as names, language, accents, religion, and various types of behavioral characteristics. In most places in the world, race and ethnicity are important issues in politics and policy decision making. They are also important criteria in the allocation of scarce resources and in personal choices concerning friendship, marriage, and place of residence. Ethnicity as well as race is a way for people to define themselves or to be defined by others; those definitions have an impact on what people are able to accomplish.

Minorities. This is a sociological term that refers to a culturally or physically distinctive social group whose members experience various disadvantages at the hands of another social group; these include prejudice, discrimination, segregation, or persecution (or a combination of these) (Vander Zanden, 1972). Where two groups are unequal in power—by virtue of superior technology or control of critical economic, political, and social institutions, the more powerful group is able to actualize its claim to an unequal and larger share of the socially defined "goods," (unless prevented by norms that restrain exploitation of the weaker by the more powerful). The social disadvantages experienced by minorities are related to their physical or cultural characteristics or both; these characteristics are held in low esteem by the dominant group. Despite its literal meaning, a minority is not a statistical category, although minority groups are generally of smaller size than the dominant group (Vander Zanden, 1972, pp. 10-11).

Prejudice. Prejudice commonly means a "prejudgment" about a person or group without bothering to verify the opinion or to examine the merits of the judgment. It involves attitudes and feelings, resulting in the tendency to engage in a negative action against the person or group for which these attitudes and feelings have developed.

Social Discrimination. This involves unfavorable treatment or action against an individual or group on the basis of ethnic or racial characteristics, gender, age, or disabilities.

Cultural Knowledge. Cultural knowledge occurs when people become familiarized with selected cultural characteristics, history, values, belief systems, and behaviors of the members of another ethnic group.

Cultural Awareness. Cultural awareness occurs when people develop sensitivity and understanding of another ethnic group. It usually involves internal changes in terms of attitudes and values. Awareness and sensitivity also refer to the qualities of openness and flexibility that people develop in relation to others. Cultural awareness must be supplemented with cultural knowledge.

Cultural Competence. Cultural or ethnic competence refers to the development of skills that will help people behave in a culturally appropriate way with a given group, demonstrating both sensitivity to cultural differences and similarities in the effective use of cultural symbols in interactions and effective communications with members of diverse populations. According to Green (1982), ethnic competence is the essential and critical characteristic of the worker who knows, appreciates, and can use the culture of another group in assisting with the resolution of a problem. To be ethnically competent means "to be able to conduct one's professional work in a way that is congruent with the behaviors and expectations that members of a distinctive culture recognize as appropriate among themselves" (Green, 1982, p. 52). It involves the acceptance of ethnic differences in a open, genuine manner, without condescension and without patronizing gestures.

Melting Pot Theory. Socialization in the United States typically includes indoctrination in the melting pot theory, which holds that American society is homogeneous. Following this belief, each new wave of immigrant groups will eventually become assimilated into one "American" culture. This theory is being challenged today, by a growing acceptance that ethnic groups are maintaining their culture and identity across generations.

Affirmative Action. This includes positive steps or legal remedies or policies to achieve equal employment and training opportunities and access to colleges and universities for women and for people of color. It is based on the notion that minorities and women should be hired and promoted in proportion to their representation in the population. It refers to steps aimed at correcting past discrimination and inequalities. Affirmative action is the process of "catching up" and integrating social and disadvantaged groups into the mainstream. It is about establishing a system of fairness.

Public resistance to affirmative action is growing (e.g., workers fear that they might be displaced by Blacks, Hispanics, or females, or by other diverse populations). This has to do with the competitive nature of the American economic system.

Quota System. The quota system refers to the establishment of a fixed, mandatory number or percentage of people to be hired or promoted, regardless of the number of potential applicants available who have the qualifications. This is contrary to numerical goals and objectives that are based on number of expected vacancies and the number of qualified applicants available. It assumes that the employer has a good faith intention to hire minorities and women.

Cultural Diversity. Cultural diversity as a concept acknowledges that we live in a society that consists of multiple groups, with each group having its own group's culture; it holds that there may be more differences among ourselves than there are similarities. The term cultural diversity conveys the message that people have the right to be different and that we need to respect that right. Cultural diversity also calls for addressing the heterogeneity and concerns of different white ethnic groups, such as Eastern Europeans, who have different languages and customs and who have continued to come to the United States.

The term cultural diversity is often used to address the special needs of racial and ethnic minorities such as Native Americans, Alaskan Natives, Asian Americans, Pacific Islanders, Hispanics/ Latinos, and African Americans, among others. In the context of this chapter, the definition of diversity extends beyond gender, racial, religious, and geographic boundaries. In its broadest form, diversity encompasses differences in culture, national origin, gender, sexual identity, socioeconomic/educational status, physical capacity (differently abled), age, language, beliefs, values, behavior patterns, or customs among the various groups within a community, organization, or nation (Giachello & Patermaster, 1994).

Diversity has received a fair amount of attention from government and corporate human services circles. Many health organizations are in the midst of a shift in addressing issues of diversity. This shift is away from addressing diversity as a legal or moral obligation (e.g., equal opportunity employment, affirmative action) to a more positive perception in which organizations look at ways in which they can value differences among staff and be more effective with their clients (Giachello & Patermaster, 1994).

Diversity has many dimensions. For women of color, this means seeking the proper balance in gender representation. In a national health organization, it includes geographic diversity (e.g., representation from Native American women living in reservations). In a direct health service agencies, it may mean the need to include women of color on boards and to accept them as clients regardless of their social and economic status and physical abilities (Houle, 1990).

Diversity also means integration, so that people's skills and ideas are used and not merely acknowledged (Morrison, 1992). For a health organization to address cultural diversity among staff, it is vital that diverse interests and characteristics within the community are reflected at all levels of the health organization.

Achieving and maintaining diversity requires organizational commitment from the top and the deliberate planning for the implementation of strategies to recruit and to retain women of color. It also requires an understanding of the breadth of diversity within a population and development of ways to identify and nurture relationships with other organizations and networks that can be a rich source for recruitment (Carver, 1993; Giachello & Patermaster, 1994).

Why Are We Concerned
With Cultural Diversity?

Several factors are responsible for our increasing interest in cultural diversity. They are related to: (a) changes in population composition, (b) new research about the disparities in health status among racial and ethnic groups, and (c) increased advocacy and activism by socially disadvantaged groups.

POPULATION GROWTH

Rapid population growth in the last decade, particularly among racial and ethnic minorities, is primarily responsible for the increased interest in culturally diverse populations. For example, from 1980 to 1990, the African American population increased by 13%, from 26.5 million to approximately 30 million; the Asian/Pacific Islander population increased 95%, from 3.7 million to 7.2 million; the number of Native Americans and Alaskan Natives increased 28%, from 1.5 million to almost 2 millions; and Hispanics/Latinos grew 53%, from 15.7 million to 22.3 million. During the same period, the "White" population increased only 5.6% (U.S. Bureau of the Census, 1993).

The growth of minority populations and the increase in U.S. immigrants have dramatically changed the face of many communities over the last decade. Health organizations are gradually expanding their services in response to these changes, and in this process meeting a series of challenges.

DISPARITIES IN DEMOGRAPHICS AND IN HEALTH STATUS

The increased interest in culturally diverse populations is also partly due to new research in the area of health, documenting the disparities in health status, health beliefs, health behaviors, and patterns of health service use.

The limited information available on women of color reveals a large disparity in their socioeconomic and demographic characteristics, compared to men and to White women. This disparity manifested itself in the areas of educational achievement, income/occupation, fertility, and health status. Each area is related to major social and structural factors that hinder women of color in developing themselves to the full extent. The need to study the health of women of color is due not only to the age structure and youthfulness of this population but also because limited studies have found that they are at highest risk for certain health conditions, such as HIV/AIDS, cancer, violence, systemic lupus, sexually transmitted diseases, diabetes, and depression, among others (NIH Office of Research on Women's Health, 1992). In addition, women of color experience a higher rate of medical indigence, and they confront a series of financial, cultural, and institutional barriers in obtaining health care. Bracho de Carpio, Carpio-Cedraro, and Anderson (1993) found that sexism, racism, and classism appeared to be the root causes of poor health status among women of color; it was not just a problem of lack of information and access to the health care system.

INCREASED POLITICAL SOPHISTICATION

The increased political sophistication and advocacy activities of groups experiencing social and economic disadvantages is a major factor responsible for the increased attention to cultural diversity. Community, grassroots, minority, and nonminority professionals have been organizing themselves more effectively and mobilizing for social action, as well as exercising their right to vote. The new technology (e.g., fax machines, E-mail, telephone conferencing) has increased communication, resulting in better networking and the development of strategies for effective change. This has led to productive discussions of and directions for critical changes within the health and human service structures. For example, due to the work of so-called radical groups such as ACT-UP, there have been meaningful changes in public policies regarding AIDS. The elderly constituency has become more vocal and politically organized, leading to a greater allocation of resources to their age peers. Groups representing people with disabilities lobbied to pass the 1993 American With Disabilities Act. Racial and ethnic minority groups have been instrumental in the passage of the Disadvantaged Minority Health Improvement Act of 1990, which includes provisions to benefit racial and ethnic groups in the area of health care.

Women's groups have also been very active. They were instrumental in the appointment of a woman for the first time ever as director of the National Institutes of Health (NIH) during 1990-1993. They also worked to establish an Office of Research on Women's Health at NIH to support behavioral and biomedical research on women of all ages.

Despite all these changes, Bracho de Carpio, Carpio-Cedraro, and Anderson (1990) found that many professionals believe that people are all alike. In their study, professionals said all people are human beings with similar life tasks and that culturally appropriate information or culturally competent staff are not necessary because universities teach standards of professional behavior that allow workers to reach clients. Bracho de Carpio et al. (1990) noted some validity in these arguments. We are all humans and have basic needs. However, the expression of those needs can be very different. Health professionals lack knowledge of the culturally expressive behaviors of their patients/clients. The health care system is a social institution that has resisted the establishment of culturally specific programs and interventions for diverse populations, as they do not perceive them to be cost-effective. The health care system prefers to continue focusing on uniformity in service delivery, for example, in appointment systems, clinic hours, and so on.

AWARENESS OF RACISM, SEXISM, AND CLASSISM

Another factor responsible for an increased interest in cultural diversity issues is the increasing public awareness of racism, sexism, classism, and social discrimination and their impact upon society's institutions.

Institutional racism refers to the established, customary, and respected ways in which society operates to keep the minority in a subordinate position (Baca Zinn, 1989). *Racism* then is any policy, practice, belief, or attitude that attributes characteristics or status to individuals based on their race, whereas *sexism* operates in a similar way based on gender (Rothenberg, 1995). Racism and sexism can be either conscious or unconscious, intentional or unintentional. Racism and sexism become institutionalized when all the institutions in society act to maintain the subordination of people of color by White people, or the subordination of women by men, and they call upon the force of history to reflect and reinforce that system of subordination and inequality (Rothenberg, 1995).

Women's groups and leaders of racial and ethnic groups seek to be viewed as equals, rather than as special interest groups or deviants from the norm, which is represented by White males or White Anglo Saxons. Institutional racism, sexism, and classicism account for many of the health and social problems of women. They are reflected in the type of policies that are developed and implemented in this country, as well as in the lack of action on behalf of disadvantaged groups and women.

Regarding women, the prevailing mentality holds that women in general are inferior to men and that their lives are not as important. Women of color, as a dual minority, are most likely to live in extreme poverty, in segregated areas (e.g. ghetto communities), in poor housing; they are most likely to be exposed to violence in the home and in the street, besides experiencing a series of health problems and social stresses. As a result, they live lives of despair, and they struggle for daily survival with limited knowledge about opportunities available to them to break this cycle. In developing this argument further, Bracho de Carpio and associates (1993) cited Knowles and Prewitt:

The institutions of society have great power to reward and penalize. They reward by providing career opportunities for some people and foreclosing them for others. They reward as well by using the way social goods and services are distributed, by deciding who receives training and skills, medical care, formal education, political influence, moral support and self-respect, productive employment, fair treatment by the law, decent housing, self-confidence and the promise of a secure future for themselves and their children. (p. 7)

Health's Initiatives for Women of Color

To address the diversity of social, economic, political, and health problems of women of color, we need to have a clear vision and understanding of their possible solutions. Most problems will take a lifetime or many generations to solve; other problems related to health care can be addressed now. This section will attempt to suggest some policies aimed at affecting the health care delivery system for women of color.

Today there is a trend toward establishing Offices for Minority Health or Women's Health in local, city, or state health departments. The purpose of these offices is to correct past institutional practices involving lack of sensitivity in addressing the diverse health needs of racial and ethnic minorities; to improve their access to the medical service system; and to promote changes in the institutional culture (i.e., values, norms, attitudes) with respect to people of color and women in the agency and beyond.

What follows is a series of policy and program recommendations that could facilitate organizational change in health services delivery to achieve diversity in reference to women. These recommendations call for commitment from top management in health organizations, recruitment of women of color in decision-making positions, and an assessment of the health needs of people of color that will lead to comprehensive health policies in the following areas:

Governance (board of directors of the organization)
Personnel
Research and planning
Community participation and input of women of color

Cultural and gender competency training

Marketing of services to women of color

Assessment of service delivery policies

Increasing/improving relationships with minority women entrepreneur/
vendors

Community prevention and education

The Evaluation or monitoring system that assesses the impact of all health
initiatives for women of color

These steps will be described in turn.

INCREASED AWARENESS AND
COMMITMENT FROM TOP MANAGEMENT

The crucial first step to address cultural diversity and the specific
needs of women of color in any health service setting (e.g., hospital,
clinics) is for the governing groups and the top management (e.g.,
president of the board, executive director/chief executive officer) to
develop an awareness and clear understanding of the rapid growth
of this population and their unique needs. Governing bodies and top
management must realize that they are operating in a dynamic environment in which, among other things, the racial/ethnic composition of
the population is changing in larger numbers. These groups have
traditionally been excluded from meaningful participation at all
levels in the health care organization. Part of this process involves an
awareness that organizations have not been as responsive to the
needs of these populations as they should have been. Recognition of
the problem by the leadership is essential for any effective action, as
well as for any organizational changes. Commitment to address
diversity issues then must be translated into policies, administrative
practices, and targeted efforts, with the proper allocation of resources
(e.g., staff and funds).

ESTABLISHMENT OF ADVISORY
GROUPS ON CULTURAL DIVERSITY

In starting a comprehensive effort to include diverse representation
of women of color, the establishment of advisory groups is crucial.
Such groups should consists of members of target populations (e.g.,

consumers, professionals, and grassroots leaders of diverse groups), people who have knowledge, credibility, and expertise regarding the ethnic/racial group(s) in question, as well as strong linkages with their communities. These groups then can exchange ideas and information about priorities and work with the organizational leadership in formulating health policies, programs, and activities based on what works and does not work for a given population, of course, considering the organization's resource limits. When these goals have been achieved, programs must be monitored to evaluate their impact.

RECRUITMENT OF WOMEN OF
COLOR IN DECISION-MAKING POSITIONS

Another strategy to achieve diversity is to recruit women of color to the Board of Directors and to high-ranking administrative decision-making positions. People in management positions can be instrumental in the development and implementation of comprehensive health policies that may lead to the implementation of culture-specific health programs. It is important to assure that people considered for these positions have a clear understanding and commitment to addressing the concerns of women of color, have social credibility, and have appropriate linkages to the community. Candidates should also have the necessary credentials and skills to do the work needed, either at the board level or in the administrative position. These people need to be supported and mentored if they are to be effective. Recruitment to leadership positions of people who reaffirm the status quo and overidentify with the institution is rarely a successful strategy for change.

ASSESSMENT OF ORGANIZATIONAL NEEDS

The fourth step, conducted simultaneously with those above, is to conduct a general needs assessment of the organization, its past and present history, problems, gaps, and strengths in addressing women of color. Several steps are suggested:

1. Board members and organizational staff involved in this initiative must become familiarized with the background (e.g., demographic, socio-economic characteristics, history) of the population(s) in question.

2. A comprehensive review of research on health services must be conducted to know the state of affairs in women's health needs and to identify the gaps in knowledge and services.

3. A comprehensive review and analysis must be made of internal documents (i.e., current policies that directly and indirectly affect women of color as clients) and of available data on women's health

4. A series of needs assessment instruments, such as a survey of staff's perceptions of agency needs and gaps in services in addressing the needs of women of color, a recurrent client satisfaction survey, and a survey of community leaders' perceptions of the agency's services and outreach efforts to women of color, should be developed and used. Focus groups with staff, clients, health care providers, and community leaders can be very useful as a substitute for and/or complement to the surveys.

Mechanisms should be established to systematically assess, on an ongoing basis, the diverse and changing needs of women of color.

Part of the organizational assessment is to examine its level of cultural competency. A typology classifying agency cultural competence on a continuum was proposed (Cross et al., 1989). The word *competence* was defined as having the capacity to function effectively. It is viewed as a goal toward which organizations should strive. Cultural competence is viewed as a developmental process. It is argued that no matter how proficient an agency may become, there will always be room for growth. Beginning with cultural destructiveness and moves to cultural proficiency, this continuum provides a useful tool by which to pinpoint possible ways of responding to cultural differences.

Cultural Destructiveness. The negative end of the continuum is represented by attitudes, policies, and practices that are destructive to cultures and consequently to the individuals within the culture. An extreme example is cultural genocide, the purposeful destruction of a culture (e.g., the systematic attempted destruction of Native American culture by the very services set up to "help" Native Americans, such as boarding schools).

Cultural Incapacity. At the next position on the continuum, the system or agencies do not intentionally seek to be culturally destructive but rather lack the capacity to help minority clients or communities. The system remains extremely biased, believes in the racial superiority of the dominant group, and assumes a paternal posture toward less powerful or "lesser" groups. Characteristics of these types of organizations include: discriminatory hiring practices, subtle messages to people of color that they are not valued or welcome, and generally lower expectations of culturally diverse clients.

Cultural Blindness. At the midpoint of the continuum, organizations provide services that express the philosophy of being unbiased. Culturally blind organizations are characterized by the belief that helping approaches traditionally used by the mainstream culture are universally applicable. These agencies encourage assimilation and blame the victims for their failures, according to the research team of (Cross et al., 1989).

Cultural Precompetence. The precompetent agency realizes its weaknesses in serving cultural diverse populations and attempts to improve some aspect of its services to specific populations. Such organizations try experiments, hire ethnic/racial staff, explore how to reach people of color in their service area, initiate training for their workers on cultural sensitivity, enter into needs assessment concerning minority communities, and recruit minority individuals for their boards of directors or advisory committees. A danger at this levels, according to (Cross et al., 1989), is a false sense of accomplishment or of failure that prevents the agency from moving forward along the continuum. Another danger is tokenism. Agencies sometime hire one or more minority workers and feel they are then equipped to meet the client's needs. Although hiring minority staff is very important, it is no guarantee that services, access, or sensitivity will be improved.

Basic Cultural Competence. At this level, organizations are characterized by acceptance and respect for difference and continuing self-assessment regarding culture differences. They work to hire unbiased staff, seek advice and consultation from members of the minority community, and actively decide what they can and cannot provide to minority clients.

Advanced Cultural Competence. Organizations operating at this level hold culture in high esteem. Such agencies seek to add to the knowledge base of culturally competent practice by conducting research and by hiring staff who are specialists in culturally competent practice. They advocate for cultural competence through the system and improve relations between cultures throughout society (Cross et al., 1989).

DEVELOPMENT OF WOMEN
OF COLOR'S HEALTH INITIATIVES

The fifth step is the development of health policies for women of color based on the needs assessment. Some suggested policy areas to be addressed are discussed below.

Personnel Policies. Policies must be developed to recruit, retain, and promote women of color at all levels in the health organizational structure. Special efforts must be made to recruit qualified women of color professionals and paraprofessionals. Clear directives must be given to top management to place a high priority on the recruitment of qualified personnel as budget allocations permit and vacancies occur. All hiring and promotions activities must be closely monitored, perhaps by any Office of Affirmative Action (although small local health departments don't have them), to assure that this will happen. Written justification should be required from administrative staff when women of color are not considered for a given position.

The following are among the strategies that can be used to identify and recruit bilingual/ bicultural staff:

Establish a community personnel recruitment advisory committee that can aggressively seek and recommend potential candidates. This advisory group should include community leaders, who are often familiar with the talent pools in their respective communities.

Conduct orientation meetings in the community to inform people on how to apply for city, state, and federal government jobs in the area of health, or how to apply to a given health organization (e.g., hospital, clinic, health maintenance organization).

Use the local and community ethnic media to announce positions in the language most often used in a given community or among selected sectors of the ethnic/racial populations.

Another strategy to consider is to provide additional monetary compensation for people who are bilingual, because of the extra work required from bilingual workers. This has proven to be effective in recruiting bilingual staff in states such as Illinois.

Within a given health facility or organization, professionals and paraprofessional must be redistributed so that bilingual and bicultural patient/clients receive services from health practitioners with bilingual and bicultural capabilities. For that purpose, an inventory or language bank of current staff with bilingual capabilities must be conducted. Part of this assessment is to explore staff interest in learning the language most often used by clients. A questionnaire can be developed to explore staff motivation and to obtain information about the level of instruction needed, beginning or intermediary. Inpatient facilities should consider creating special units when there is an adequate concentration of clients and staff.

Incentives are needed to retain staff who are women of color. Part of this process can include the development and implementation of management development internship programs and tuition reimbursement for undergraduate and graduate education to enhance the knowledge and skill levels that prepare these workers for managerial positions. Mentoring should be used to support new staff and consultants when they must work in relative isolation.

The reasons for the departure of women of color staff need to be assessed. The institution should review its reward systems and how it welcomes and integrates minority women staff. New methods of strengthening the commitment of these workers to the agency should be considered.

Research and Planning. Because of the uniqueness and changing needs of women of color, and the limited health data available, ongoing research, planning, and evaluation services are needed. In this process, it is essential to generate, publish, and disseminate health data on women of color useful for program planning and development and for public policy formulation. These initiatives are important because in our times hard data are needed to justify allocation of resources and to influence plans regarding sites for facilities, need for bilingual staff, and so on. Some of the suggested strategies involve the following:

Modify data forms to include identifiers of Latino, Asian, and Native American subpopulations, as well as national origins.

Allocate resources (funds and staff) for research, planning, and evaluation. This will ensure that the proper changes in collection and data analysis can take place, leading to the generation and publication of reports, for example, in the area of vital statistics.

Conduct ongoing needs assessment studies (i.e., patient satisfaction surveys, etc.). These investigations may lead to the development of comprehensive health and mental health programs and specialized services for women of color and/or improvement of the service delivery components.

Another purpose of research and planning policy is to form new partnerships. These can take place with local universities for conjoint research projects and with community groups or city, county, and state agencies that may be interested in conducting research on the health of women of color. Technical assistance should be sought from universities on how to conduct community surveys, data management and analyses, and other research activities. Women of color researchers should be part of any research effort to assure that the formulation of the problem, instrument development, and data collection and analysis will be done within an appropriate cultural framework. This will minimize the negative stereotypes that have been generated by nonminority researchers with limited knowledge of women of color.

Finally, needs assessment and research findings should be shared with community leaders, service providers, and policymakers so they can engage in better program planning and be able to advocate effectively for services in their communities.

Community Participation and Input. Because public and private health organizations have not traditionally worked closely with minority organizations, distrustful attitudes often develop when people begin to work together. To develop meaningful partnerships and trustful relations with communities of color, and to assure that their health and social needs are taken into consideration, city and state health departments and health organizations in the private sector must seek involvement and input by women of color as they develop policies and programs that will have a direct or indirect impact on have a direct or indirect impact on these women's lives. At the community level, this can be accomplished through participation by women of color on advisory groups for health facilities, as well as by holding community dialogue meetings. The advisory groups can assist in (a) assessment of community health and social needs, (b) outreach efforts and health marketing of the services to the community, and (c) assessment of current community perceptions of the delivery of health services. These boards should represent both consumers' and providers' interests. Special efforts must be made to engage in contractual agreements with community-based organizations serving women of color to coordinate efforts for the delivery of certain health or mental health services.

Marketing of Services to Women of Color. The main aim of this policy is to increase awareness of the agency's services and activities among women of color, while changing some of the negative community perceptions of the health organization. In implementing this policy, women of color without a regular source of care can be identified and linked to existing health resources. Outreach efforts, particularly in areas with high concentrations of women of color, must be pursued. This can be accomplished through extensive marketing of health care and mental health services and through the use of outreach workers or "health promoters." The media can also play a critical role in informing the community of the health resources available, location of services, procedures to follow to receive services, and their cost. Some activities may call for an increased participation in radio, TV, and cable talk shows; preparation of columns and press releases for community papers, targeting communities of color; and establishment of a bilingual speakers' bureau. The development and distribution of a bilingual health bulletin can also increase awareness of service availability to non-English speaking minority populations.

Assessment of an In-House Health Delivery Policy and System. As a means of making health services more accessible and relevant to women of color, the health facility must examine its service delivery policies to make them accessible and affordable. This requires assessing the appointment system, walk-in policies, cost of care, protocol for use of interpreters, and hours of services. Agencies need to explore ways of reducing the length of time between making an appointment and the actual visit to the facility, as well as clients' waiting time once they come to the facility. Criteria and eligibility requirements for the delivery of services should also be examined. Culturally insensitive policies and procedures must be identified, and strategies for change must be developed.

In-Service Training on Cultural Awareness. Ongoing culturally specific, in-service training programs must be designed and implemented for staff at all levels in the department. These training sessions must be geared toward developing knowledge, awareness, and sensitivity of everything that affects the health of women of color: socioeconomic and demographic factors, health beliefs, health status, migration patterns, family systems, religion, health behaviors, and other cultural factors. These sessions should be ongoing and should be used to assist staff in examining their attitudes, prejudices, and behaviors toward minority women clients. Staff should have the opportunity to share with each other their experiences and frustrations in dealing with people about whom they know very little and with whom communication is often difficult. The ultimate goal is to help staff to develop cultural and gender-specific competence.

Community Health Education. Finally, policies addressing community health education activities must be a part of this comprehensive model to address the health needs of women of color. Several suggestions include the following:

> Establish health promotion or wellness centers or programs.
> Develop bilingual educational materials (an inventory of existing materials must first be conducted to identify gaps),
> Implement health education activities in the community at appropriate reading levels, using nontraditional models such as the home "Tupperware party."
> Participate in community activities such as health fairs and other community events (i.e., school immunization campaign).

Participation in community activities allows organizations to improve their image, facilitate informal communication with leaders, and spread the word on the kinds of activities they are doing on behalf of women of color. It also serves as a means of becoming acquainted with communities of color. Community groups are appreciative when representatives from health organizations attend their social events.

Health education activities should focus on the following priority areas based on community perceptions, which are not always in concordance with epidemiological indicators:

Maternal and child care because of the high fertility of women of color and the many health problems that affect poor minority women and children

Violence

Health maintenance and health promotion

Mental health

Alcohol and substance abuse issues

HIV/AIDS and other sexually-transmitted diseases

Minority Women Contractor/Vendors. Because health care is a big industry that generates jobs and contracts, any health care delivery system committed to addressing the health needs of women of color should be open to increasing the pool of minority women-owned businesses and consultants it uses. The organization should assess its current linkages and number of contracts with minority populations and with women and should provide technical assistance and training so they can compete successfully for service contracts and grants.

Finally, in order to implement health policies aimed at women of color, it is important to inform and educate agency staff at all levels about why is it important to address the health needs of women of color, and to involve staff at all levels at all stages of the process (from planning to implementation). Otherwise they may experience fears and insecurities; they may think that "now women of color are taking over." Therefore, clear and open communication with staff is necessary and extremely important. Through active staff input, participation, and teamwork, it will be possible to obtain the cooperation necessary for a successful implementation of health policies.

Summary

There has been a rapid increase in the number and diversity of women of color across the nation. In small towns, rural areas, and big cities, their poor health status relative to whites has been well documented. Health organizations at the local and national levels, whether or not they are service delivery, must develop and implement health policies to address the diverse health needs of women of color in a comprehensive manner. The Cultural Competency Continum helps in assessing where the organization stands in this area. Past institutional practices should be corrected, and the culture (i.e., norms, values, behaviors) that prevail in the health care system must change. Suggested steps, strategies, and policy areas to be addressed have been set forth in this chapter.

References

Baca Zinn, M. (1989). Problems of inequality: Race and ethnicity. In D. Stanley & M. Baca Zinn (Eds.), *Social problems (4th ed.*, pp.132-149). Needham Heights, MA: Allyn & Bacon.

Bracho de Carpio, A., Carpio-Cedraro, F., & Anderson, L. (1990). Hispanic families learning and teaching about AIDS: A participatory approach at the community level. *Hispanic Journal of Behavioral Sciences, 12*(2), 165-176.

Bracho de Carpio, A., Carpio-Cedraro, F., & Anderson, L. (1993, September). *Latino female poverty and HIV prevention: An overspoken and undeveloped link.* Paper presented at UCLA Latino Health Research Conference, Los Angeles.

Carver, J. (1993, July-August). Achieving meaningful diversity in the board room. *Board Leadership, 8,* 287-302.

Cross, T. L., Bazrou, B. J., Dennis, L. W., & Isaacs, M. R. (1989). Washington, DC: CASSP Technical Assistance Center, Georgetown University Child Development Center.

Disadvantaged Minority Health Improvement Act of 1990, Public Law No. 101-527.

Feagin, J. R. (1989). *Racial and ethnic relations* (3rd ed.). Englewood Cliffs, NJ: Prentice Hall.

Giachello, A., & Patermaster, M. (1994). *Knowledge, attitudes, and behaviors of board of directors of nonprofit organizations about culturally diversity issues: Summary of findings of focus groups and national survey.* Unpublished report submitted to the National Center for Nonprofit Boards, Washington, DC, 1994.

Green, J. W. (1982). *Cultural awareness in the human services.* Englewood Cliffs, NJ: Prentice Hall.

Houle, C. O. (1990, January/February). Who should be on your board? *Nonprofit World, 8.*

Morrison, A. (1992). *The new leaders: Guidelines on leadership development in America*. San
    Francisco: Jossey-Bass.
Office of Research on Women's Health. (1992). *National Institutes of Health: Opportunities for Research on Women's Health*. Hunt Valley, MD: Author.
Rothenberg, P. S. (1995). *Race, class, and gender in the United States: An integrated study* (3rd ed.). New York: St. Martin's.
U.S. Bureau of the Census. (1993). *The Hispanic population in the United States: March, 1993* (CPR No. 475). Washington, DC: Government Printing Office.
Vander Zanden, J. (1972). *American minority relations* (3rd ed.). New York: The Ronald Press.

3 Native American Women's Health Concerns

Toward Restoration of Harmony

LILLIAN TOM-ORME

The health of Native American men and women continues to deteriorate in the 1990s, due to multiple causes. Until the 1950s, Native Americans died from epidemics of infectious diseases such as tuberculosis, measles, and smallpox; today, they are suffering from chronic diseases and social illnesses. The health status of Native American women is of particular concern today. Native American women, who are considered to be the central caregivers or backbone of the Indian family and kin networks, suffer disproportionately from various health problems that are considered to be preventable. These health problems have social, cultural, economic, and political implications.

This chapter will briefly outline the status of Native American women's health and suggest some ways to regain health and restore the harmony that is much revered by Native American communities. This chapter will also document the health needs of women and will include the author's personal experiences as a Native American woman, caregiver, and health care professional. The terms *American Indians/Alaskan Natives* and *Native Americans* will be used interchangeably to refer to indigenous people of the continental United States and Alaska.

The Indian Health Service (IHS) literature refers to American Indian/Alaskan Natives, whereas social science literature uses the term Native American. Either is acceptable. Readers are cautioned that where specific rates of health problems among females are absent, references will be made to the general Indian population. Note, too, that studies often vary by methodology, geographic region, and tribe; there are also differences between urban and reservation-based populations.

According to the 1990 census, the American Indian/Alaskan Native (AI/AN) population consists of over 1.9 million people, less than 2% of the total U.S. population. The Native American population in the United States comprises an estimated 400 tribal nations, speaking about 200 languages or dialects. The term *nations* is used here to refer to the original treaties made between sovereign powers (Indians and the U.S. government). Over one half of Native Americans are female, and over one half are 24 years old or younger (IHS, 1989). Approximately 55% of Native Americans reside in urban areas, and the remainder live on reservations throughout the country. Many people move off the reservation to seek employment and education or to find a different way of life outside the reservation setting. However, many who venture away from their homelands find themselves deeper in poverty. They also are more likely to suffer ill health due to lack of access to health care or employment, because they lack the skills to adapt to the demanding urban environment.

The IHS, a branch of the U.S. Public Health Service, provides health care services to American Indians and Alaskan Natives. This responsibility is specified in the U.S. Constitution (IHS, 1989). The IHS provides services to members of federally recognized tribes residing on reservations and to some urban populations. Those who may not be eligible for IHS-funded care are members of nonrecognized tribes, people with employment benefits, or those who have voluntarily broken ties with their tribe or reservation. Close to 50% of urban native women reported a household income of $10,000, compared to 15% of white women; about half of Indian women reported having some type of insurance coverage, but they were less likely to have Medicaid than their white or African American counterparts (Sugarman, Brenneman, LaRoque, Warren, & Goldberg, 1994).

The leading causes of death among Native American women include heart diseases (22.1%), malignant neoplasms (16.3%), injuries (5.7%), cerebrovascular diseases, diabetes mellitus (5.7%), and chronic liver disease and cirrhosis (IHS, 1989).

Heart Disease

Among both Native American men and women, heart disease has replaced accidents as the leading cause of death over the past few years. In a multitribe prospective study of cardiovascular disease (CVD), Welty (1992) found that between 30% and 40% of all Indian study participants had a cholesterol level of at least 200 mg/dl. Low density lipoprotein levels and smoking rates were highest among Northern Plains tribes (40% to 58%) and lowest among Southwestern tribes.

A study of Navajos in the Southwest found that 17.5% of women in the sample had cholesterol concentrations equal to or greater than 240 mg/dl, compared to 32.7% of women from the general population (Sugarman, Gilbert, Percy, & Peter, 1992). Although Navajo women show lower cholesterol concentrations, increases will most likely occur soon. Obesity as a risk factor for chronic diseases is extremely common—up to 68% of Indian people are obese. The mean body mass index (BMI) of Plains women is at least 30 (Newman, Hollevoet, & Fohlich, 1993; Welty, 1992). Among Northern Ute women with diabetes, the mean BMI of women was 57 (Tom-Orme, 1988).

A 1987 survey of American Indian and Alaskan Native people 19 years or older revealed that 22% of females reported having high blood pressure, compared to 23% of females in the general U.S. population (National Center for Health Statistics, 1990, p. 28). Hypertension is generally found in approximately one half of the diabetic population. Among Native Americans, diabetic hypertension is estimated to be from 30% to 50% (IHS, 1989). Thus, hypertension rates among Native American women are comparable to women in the general population.

Among a small sample of urban American Indians, cardiovascular and stroke risk factors, such as cigarette smoking (70%), diabetes (10%), and obesity, were found to be more prevalent than among whites (Gillum, Gillum, & Smith, 1984). Rates for females were not specified in this study. Among Southwestern tribes such as the Navajo, heart disease was once considered rare (Page, Lewis, & Gilbert, 1956). However, with increasing rates of tobacco use, obesity, diabetes, and hypertension, the gap between cholesterol concentrations among the Navajo and the general population has narrowed (Sugarman, Gilbert, Percy, et al., 1992). Again, rates for females were not specified; but Navajo women, in general, have lower rates than other Indian women but higher rates than white women.

Cancer

According to the New Mexico Tumor Registry, American Indian women living in New Mexico and Arizona have a cervical cancer incidence of 20.5 per 100,000 population, a rate two times greater than the rate for white females, which is 8.6 per 100,000 (Burhansstipanov & Dressler, 1993). Between 1974 and 1976, the IHS documented cervical cancer mortality to be 2.29 times greater in Native American women. The New Mexico Tumor Registry documented a 25.8% mortality rate for Native American women, compared to 10.2% for white and 12.5% for Hispanic women in New Mexico. Rates for other ethnic women were not documented in this study, probably due to small numbers of other ethnic women in this region.

Jordan and Key (1981) found that the majority of in situ and invasive cancer found in New Mexico and Arizona American Indian women occurred in women over age 60. Once Indian women reached age 30, the rate of cervical screening declined steadily. Some reasons found for this decline in screening were failure to return for follow-up clinic visits, difficulty in locating women living in isolated areas, and the highly mobile lifestyle of these women.

Other reasons identified elsewhere are the beliefs of Southwest Indian women that female health examinations are necessary only during the childbearing years and their fear of being told of abnormal results (Tom-Orme, 1993). Additional reasons for low levels of screening are the emphasis on acute care rather than preventive care and the perception by women that cancer is less serious than the pervasive conditions of diabetes and alcoholism (Tom-Orme, 1993).

The cervical cancer mortality rate of 12.5 among Alaskan Native women between 1977 and 1983 was higher than that of any other group of American Indian females (Burhansstipanov & Dressler, 1993). During this same period, the overall rate for American Indian women was 5.5, exceeding the rate of 3.2 in white women. The 5-year cancer survival rate for American Indian women is 65.1%, second only to African American women at 61.3% (Burhansstipanov & Dressler, 1993).

BREAST CANCER

In general, American Indian women have a lower incidence of breast cancer (21.7/100,000) than white women (93.3/100,000) in the United Sates (Burhansstipanov & Dressler, 1993). However, there may be variations in incidence by region and, perhaps, tribal membership. For example, Alaskan Native women have breast cancer incidence of 44.2, whereas Athapaskan Native women have an age-adjusted rate comparable to the U.S. female population (Burhansstipanov & Dressler, 1993).

Although breast cancer morbidity is generally lower for American Indian women, compared to other ethnic or racial groups, the survival rate is poor, indicating that breast cancer is diagnosed at later stages in Indian women (Burhansstipanov & Dressler, 1993). Age-adjusted breast cancer mortality rates among American Indian (9.0/100,000) and Alaskan Native women (12.8/100,000) are lower than rates for white women (26.7/100,000). However, this may be due to racial misclassification on death certificates (Burhansstipanov & Dressler, 1993).

LUNG CANCER

The incidence of lung cancer is generally low among Southwestern Indian women (a range of 4.1 to 17.9/100,000) but dramatically higher in non-Southwestern Indian women (a range of 10.3 to 111.3/100,000)

(Burhansstipanov & Dressler, 1993). The highest rates are found in Alaskan Natives, Eskimos, and Northern Plains women from the IHS service areas of Billings and Bemidji (Burhansstipanov & Dressler, 1993); these incidence rates exceed those of white women (36.3/100,000) from New Mexico.

Smoking patterns and rates among Native Americans vary by tribe, region, and other characteristics (Rhoades, Reyes, & Buzzard, 1987; Welty, 1992). Navajos have a smoking incidence of about 13% whereas Oklahoma Indians are reported to have smoking and lung cancer rates that are similar to the national rate (Rhoades et al., 1987). Furthermore, Northern Plains tribes have smoking rates between 40% and 58% (Welty, 1992; Welty, Zephier, Schweigman, Blake, & Leonardson, 1993). In a study of urban Native American clinic users in four U.S. urban settings, Native American smokers reported a median daily consumption of 11 cigarettes, compared to 20 cigarettes in the general population (Lando, Johnson, Graham-Tomasi, McGovern, & Solberg, 1992). Smoking rates are not commonly documented by gender. In a study among Montana Indian women, 50% of on-reservation as compared to 62% of off-reservation residents were smokers (Goldberg et al., 1991). It is estimated that the current smoking rate is 31% for all American Indian females (National Center for Health Statistics, 1990, p. 30). Smoking among pregnant Indian women is a serious concern. Davis, Helgerson, and Waller (1992) found that, when adjusted for maternal age and marital status, smoking rates among pregnant Indian women exceeded those of white women, 34.2 and 25.9, respectively. Northern Plains tribes are considered to have the highest cigarette smoking rate, which may be attributed to tobacco use in their cultural and religious practices. Reduction of smoking rates to achieve the Healthy People Year 2000 Objectives of 20% may be more difficult among Northern Plains women.

The use of smokeless tobacco among American Indian/Alaskan Native females is an increasing problem in all age groups. Native American women over the age of 18 were reported to use smokeless tobacco more than any other racial group in a sample surveyed by the Centers for Disease Control ("Childbearing Patterns," 1993). In a review of nine studies, which included findings from the Behavioral Risk Factor Surveillance System (BRFSS) among Native American populations, Bruerd (1990) reported that alarming rates of regular smokeless tobacco use were reported by all kindergartners (13% to 21%) surveyed, and specifically by 23% to 45% of kindergarten girls. In another study, 68.9% of sixth-grade Native American girls from IHS sites reported experimenting with smokeless tobacco, compared to 8.7% of girls from non-IHS sites (Backinger, Bruerd, Kinney, & Szpuner, 1993). Smokeless tobacco use varies by tribe and region, but it is consistently higher in Indian females than in the general female population.

Diabetes

Non-insulin dependent diabetes (NIDDM) has had ravaging effects on indigenous U.S. populations for the past 50 years. The prevalence of diabetes varies by tribe and region. The Pima Indians of south-central Arizona are reported to have the highest prevalence in the world, with 50% of their adult population (35 and older) diagnosed with diabetes (Sievers & Fisher, 1985). Drastic changes in lifestyle, such as increased sedentary activity, greater access to and consumption of high-fat foods, and obesity, seem to contribute extensively to this devastating health problem. NIDDM in Native American peoples seems to be the same condition that affects the general population.

Studies specific to Indian women are few; however, studies that mention women report higher prevalence or higher numbers of women clinic users. Although Navajo women of the Southwest tend to have lower rates than other tribes, their age-adjusted prevalence of 18.4% is 2.5 times greater than that in the general population (Sugarman, Gilbert, & Weiss, 1992).

Brosseau (1993) reported that in 1988, 65% of Fort Berthold patients found to have diabetes were women; this figure was more than double the rate observed between 1975 and 1988 in the same population. Between 1980 and 1985, an intervention among the Northern Ute tribe documented that 61% of the total diabetic population was female (Tom-Orme, 1988).

Although characteristics of diabetes are the same for Native Americans as for their white counterparts, sociocultural factors complicate diabetes management among Native Americans. People with diabetes have reported that the illness causes suffering not only for them as individuals but also for their families and communities (Tom-Orme, 1988). Brosseau (1993) identified racism, stereotyping, and cultural conflict as adding to the challenges faced by health care professionals who work with Native American populations. Thus diabetes is more than a biophysiological event.

Obesity is a major contributor to diabetes development. Leonard, Wilson, and Leonard (1986) reported that 55% of women ages 21 to 40 years old and two thirds of adult women over age 40 who participated in a community screening were obese. In a study of fifth-grade Pueblo and Navajo students, one third had BMI values indicating obesity (Davis et al., 1992). The latter study suggests that these children will become obese adults, a finding that challenges health care providers to design child-focused interventions. Community-based exercise programs have been demonstrated to be effective in weight loss and glucose control in those with diabetes (Heath, Leonard, Wilson, Kendrick, & Powell, 1987). This approach is also good in Indian communities that emphasize close-knit interactions and extended kinship ties.

Intentional and Nonintentional Injuries

In 1986, the mortality due to vehicular crashes and accidents among Indian populations was 83.2/100,000, compared to a rate in the general U.S. population of 35.2/100,000 (IHS, 1989). Among Indian females under age 5 and 25 to 54 years of age, motor vehicle crashes caused more than 2.5 times as many deaths as among the general population. Similarly, deaths from other accidents remain generally higher than among the general population, and deaths were two times greater for age groups under 1 and 15-64 years old.

Using the BRFSS data among Native Americans, Sugarman, Warren, Oge, and Helgerson (1992) found that 72.7% of women from the Plains states reported not using seat belts, compared to 17.9% of women from the West Coast states. These rates exceeded objectives of The Healthy People 2000 objectives, which are to decrease seat belt nonuse to less than 15%. Reasons for nonuse of seat belts were not given, but the sparsity of population and traffic in the Plains states may be a factor in determining whether a seat belt is used.

Alcoholism

Native American women consider alcoholism to be the leading health problem among the general Indian population (Tom-Orme, 1993). Alcohol use during pregnancy is of particular concern, due to its association with fetal alcohol syndrome (FAS). A study among the Northern Plains Indians postulated an FAS rate of 8.5 cases per 1,000 live births (Duimstra, Johnson, Kutsch, Wang, & Zentner, 1993). Further studies are needed in this area. Mortality due to alcoholism among 45-64-year-old Native American women is 54 per 100,000, compared to 8 per 100,000 for white women. According to the IHS, mortality from alcoholism decreased from 54.5 per 100,000 in 1976 to 26.1 in 1985; however, a four-fold difference still exists between Indians and the general population (Rhoades, Mason, Eddy, Smith, & Burn, 1988). In 1985, a 50-step strategic plan was developed by the IHS for prevention and health promotion programs to target school-age children, including those in Head Start; prenatal clients; adults in treatment programs; and Indian communities. Some tribes have passed resolutions through their governing bodies to combat alcoholism (Rhoades et al., 1988). Besides contributing to physical health effects, alcohol and drug abuse may also account for the rising incidence of domestic violence, including spousal, child, and elder abuse.

Domestic Violence

Domestic violence among Native Americans is an increasing and serious problem, although documentation remains scanty. The increasing incidence of spouse abuse, primarily wife abuse, is attributed to social services systems that do not recognize the problem, the deterioration of the traditional family structure, alcoholism, and the lingering effects of historical oppression (Wilson, Thomann, & Gish, 1993). Additional contributing factors include unemployment or underemployment, cultural acceptance of wife beating, availability of weapons, media portrayal of violence as entertainment, disrupted families, overcrowded and substandard housing, discrimination, lack of adequate support systems, and reluctance to seek help. In other words, the problem is multifaceted and complicated, requiring the cooperation of varied helping agencies and professionals, as well as native populations themselves. Durst (1991) found that in Arctic native traditions, chiefs intervened through communitarianism to re-solve conjugal violence. A privatized response, frequently used today, involves avoidance; this creates feelings of frustration, helplessness, and social isolation on the part of the abused as well as the community.

In 1988, the United States recorded a homicide rate of 9.0/100,000, a rate three to eight times higher than most industrialized nations (National Center for Health Statistics, 1990, p. 17). Violence in Indian communities is an ever increasing concern. Although the use of handguns by American Indians was reported to be 29% in 1988, the use of knives and stabbing accounted for 32% of the reported violence. Although the number of violent acts was lower among American Indians than among other racial groups (a range of 47% to 51%), it nonetheless is a disconcerting problem.

Elder abuse is suspected by health care providers, as well as social service providers, but there are few data. During fieldwork in 1994, the author observed that elderly people are increasingly sent to nursing homes or abandoned by adult children who seek employment away from traditional family homes, perhaps as a result of changing societal norms, such as the shifting of extended family households.

Studies of elder abuse are extremely few, focusing primarily on white women; similar studies are needed among women of color. Factors such as the changing family structure, financial difficulties, physical limitations, and emotional burden may contribute to elder abuse (Wilson et al., 1993). Native American communities are concerned about the increasing neglect of elders, but resources seem to be limited to deal with them (personal observation).

Mental health problems affecting Native American women are poorly documented. Women between the ages of 15 and 34 have a suicide rate of 9/100,000, almost twice the rate of 5/100,000 in white women. Studies of children show that 23% of boarding school students report attempted suicide (Manson, Beals, Dick, & Duclos, 1989), at least 60% of adolescents were abused or neglected (Lujan, DeBruyn, May, & Bird, 1989; Piasecki et al., 1989), and alcohol abuse was present in about 85% of neglect cases and 63% of abuse cases reported. These studies suggest intergenerational perpetuation of pathological family dynamics and calls for preventive strategies in children. Studies are needed among both Native American women, and women in general.

Birthrates and Maternal Health Status

According to the Centers for Disease Control and Prevention, between 1980 and 1990, the Native American population grew by 38%, a high rate but one somewhat lower than other ethnic groups. Between 1984 and 1986, the IHS reported the AI/AN birthrate to be 28/1,000 population, 79% greater than the rate of 15.6 in the general population (IHS, 1989). Thus the Native American population is growing rapidly, at an average rate of 3% annually. The average number of children per Native American woman ranged from 2.2 to 2.5 in 1990.

In 1990 American Indian and Alaskan Native women (53.6) ranked third compared to African American (66.7) and Cuban American (55.9) women in the percentage of births to unmarried mothers ("Childbearing Patterns," 1993). In about 19.5% of AI/AN births, the mothers are teenagers, a rate that is approximately twice the white teenage birthrate ("Childbearing Patterns," 1993). Teen pregnancies may not simply reflect the poverty of subpopulations; they also may result from more complex ingredients of low income, poor education systems, and political and cultural factors. Additional contributors are the lack of available family planning programs, support systems or services, access to general health care, health coverage, and culturally acceptable prenatal health services.

Rates of low birth weight (LBW) were 6% to 7%, despite the fact that Native American infants are considered to be at high risk for infant morbidity and mortality ("Childbearing Patterns," 1993). LBW is attributed to fetal alcohol syndrome (FAS), assisted ventilation births to mothers less than 20 years of age, higher rates of tobacco use, and other health problems, such as diabetes, obesity, and hypertension ("Childbearing Patterns," 1993). Infant deaths attributable to maternal smoking were estimated to be 16.6% in the Northern Plains, 16.2% in Alaska, and 5.2% in the Southwest (Bulterys, 1990). The incidence of sudden infant death syndrome is over three times greater among Northern Plains Indians and Alaskan Natives (4.6 per 1,000 live births) than among Southwestern Indians (1.4 per 1,000 live births); the higher incidence is attributed to maternal smoking (Bulterys, 1990).

Infectious Diseases

Tuberculosis (TB) rates have increased throughout the country since about 1985, due to the influx of foreign-born people from TB-endemic areas, the HIV/AIDS epidemic, poverty and homelessness, deteriorating public infrastructure, and lack of concern by providers. In Native Americans, tuberculosis rates have decreased dramatically; however, the incidence is five times higher in Native American females (11.4 per 100,000) than in white women (2.4 per 100,000), according to the Centers for Disease Control (1993). The HIV seroprevalence is similar among rural and urban American Indian women, indicating spread of HIV from urban to rural populations. In addition, HIV rates among third-trimester Native American women in three Western states were four to eight times higher than women of other races in the same states (Conway et al., 1992).

Summary

Native American women suffer from poor health despite the availability of health care services through the IHS, the major health care provider. Although great strides have been made by the IHS in providing direct health care and environmental health services (Rhoades et al., 1987), women are experiencing higher rates of diabetes and related problems, domestic violence, lung cancer, tobacco use, obesity, cervical cancer, and problems related to childbearing. Many health problems specific to Native American women are poorly documented.

Some recommendations to improving the health status of American Indian and Alaskan Native women are as follows:

1. Involve women in their personal health care to prevent further problems and promote healthy practices.

2. Increase the involvement of women in planning and participation in the involvement of community-level interventions, particularly in regions where higher rates of health problems are found.

3. Ensure that health care services are culturally competent to meet the specific needs of women by tribe or region.

4. Create more opportunities for local training of providers so that ancillary staff will be more aware of local needs, beliefs, attitudes, and practices that would promote greater cooperation and participation by tribes and communities.

5. Promote educational opportunities to students at all levels to increase the number of indigenous health care professionals in tribal communities.

References

Backinger, C. L., Bruerd, B., Kinney, M. B., & Szpuner, S. M. (1993). Knowledge, intent to use, of smokeless tobacco among sixth grade school children in six selected U.S. sites. *Public Health Reports, 8*(5), 637-642.

Brosseau, J. D. (1993). Diabetes and Indians. In J. R. Joe & R. S. Young (Eds.), *Diabetes as a disease of civilization: The impact of culture change on indigenous peoples* (pp. 41-66). New York: Mouton de Gruyter.

Bruerd, B. (1990). Smokeless tobacco use among Native American school children. *Public Health Reports, 105*(2), 196-201.

Bulterys, M. (1990). High incidence of sudden infant death syndrome among Northern Indians and Alaska Natives compared with Southwestern Indians: Possible role of smoking. *Journal of Community Health, 15*(3), 185-194.

Burhansstipanov, L., & Dressler, C. M. (1993). *Native American monograph No. 1: Documentation of the cancer research needs of American Indian and Alaskan Native* (NIH Publication No. 93-3603). Washington, DC: National Institute of Cancer.

Centers for Disease Control. (1993). *Reported tuberculosis in the United States, 1993.* Atlanta: Author.

Childbearing patterns among selected racial/ethnic minority groups—United States, 1990. (1993, May 28). *Morbidity and Mortality Weekly Report,* pp. 398-403.

Conway, G. A., Ambrose, T. J., Chase, E., Hooper, E. Y., Helgerson, S. D., Johannes, P., Epstein, M. R., McRae, B. A., Munn, V. P., & Keevama, L. (1992). HIV infection in American Indians and Alaskan Natives: Surveys in the Indian Health Service. *Journal of Acquired Immune Deficiency Syndrome, 5*(8), 803-809.

Davis, R. L., Helgerson, S. D., & Waller, P. (1992). Smoking during pregnancy among northwest Native Americans. *Public Health Reports, 107*(1), 66-69.

Duimstra, C., Johnson, D., Kutsch, C., Wang, B., & Zentner, M. (1993). A fetal alcohol syndrome surveillance pilot project in American Indian communities in the Northern Plains. *Public Health Reports, 108*(2), 225-229.

Durst, D. (1991). Conjugal violence: Changing attitudes in two northern native communities. *Community Mental Health Journal, 27*(5), 359-372.

Gillum, R. F., Gillum, B. S., & Smith, N. (1984). Cardiovascular risk factors among urban American Indians: Blood pressure, serum lipids, smoking, diabetes, health knowledge, and behavior. *American Heart Journal, 107,* 765-776.

Goldberg, H. I., Warren, C. W., Oge, L. L., Helgerson, S. D., Pepion, D. D., LaMere, E., & Friedman, J. S. (1991). Prevalence of behavioral risk factors in two American Indian populations in Montana. *American Journal of Preventive Medicine, 7*(3), 155-160.

Heath, G. W., Leonard, B. E., Wilson, R. H., Kendrick, J. S., & Powell, K. E. (1987). Community-based exercise intervention: Zuni diabetes project. *Diabetes Care, 10*(5), 579-583.

Indian Health Service. (1989). *Trends in Indian health care* (U.S. DHHS Publication). Washington, DC: Author.

Jordan, S. W., & Key, C. R. (1981). Carcinoma of the cervix in southwestern American Indians: A result of a cytologic detection program. *Cancer, 47*(29), 2523-2532.

Lando, H. A., Johnson, K. M., Graham-Tomasi, R. P., McGovern, P. G., & Solberg, L. (1992). Urban Indians' smoking patterns and interest in quitting. *Public Health Reports, 107*(3), 340-344.

Leonard, B., Wilson, R., & Leonard, C. (1986). Zuni diabetes project. *Public Health Reports, 101,* 282-288.

Lujan, C., DeBruyn, L. M., May, P. A., & Bird, M. E. (1989). Profile of abused and neglected American Indian children in the Southwest. *Child Abuse & Neglect, 13*(4), 449-461.

Manson, S. M., Beals, J., Dick, R. W., & Duclos, C. (1989). Risk factors for suicide among Indian adolescents at a boarding school. *Public Health Reports, 104*(6), 609-614.

National Center for Health Statistics. (1990). *Health United States 1990* (U.S. DHHS Publication No. 91-1232). Hyattsville, MD: Author.

Newman, W. P., Hollevoet, J. J., & Fohlich, K. L. (1993). The diabetes project at Fort Totten, North Dakota, 1984-1983. *Diabetes Care, 16*(1), 361-363.

Page, I. H., Lewis, L. A., & Gilbert, J. (1956). Plasma lipids and proteins and their relationship to coronary disease among Navajo Indians. *Circulation, 13,* 675-679.

Piasecki, J. M., Manson, S. M., Biernoff, M. P., Hiat, A. B., Taylor, S. S., & Bechtol, D. W. (1989). Abuse and neglect of American Indian children: Findings from a survey of federal providers. *American Indian/Alaskan Natives Mental Health Research, 3*(2), 43-62.

Rhoades, E. R., Mason, R. D., Eddy, P., Smith, E. M., & Burn, T. R. (1988). The Indian Health Service approach to alcoholism among American Indians and Alaskan Natives. *Public Health Reports, 103*(6), 621-627.

Rhoades, E. R., Reyes, L. L., & Buzzard, G. D. (1987). The organization of health services for Indian people. *Public Health Reports, 102*(4), 352-356.

Sievers, M. L., & Fisher, J. R. (1985). Diabetes in North American Indians. In M. I. Harris & R. F. Hamman (Eds.), *Diabetes in America* (Chapter 11). Rockville, MD: U.S. DHHS.

Sugarman, J. R., Brenneman, G., LaRoque, L., Warren, C. W., and Goldberg, H. I. (1994). The urban American Indian oversample in the 1988 national maternal and infant health survey. *Public Health Reports, 109*(2), 243-250.

Sugarman, J. R., Gilbert, T. J., Percy, C. A., & Peter, D. A. (1992). Serum cholesterol concentrations among Navajo Indians. *Public Health Reports, 107*(1), 92-99.

Sugarman, J. R., Gilbert, T. J., & Weiss, N. S. (1992). Prevalence of diabetes and impaired glucose tolerance among Navajo Indians. *Diabetes Care, 15*(1), 114-120.

Sugarman, J. R., Warren, C. W., Oge, L., & Helgerson, S. D. (1992). Using the behavioral risk factor surveillance system to monitor year 2000 objectives among American Indians. *Public Health Reports, 107*, 449-456.

Tom-Orme, L. (1988). Chronic disease and the social matrix: A Native American diabetes intervention. *Recent Advances in Nursing, 22*, 89-109.

Tom-Orme, L. (1993, September). *Breast and cervical cancer knowledge, attitudes, and beliefs of Native American women: Findings from focus group interviews.* Paper presented at the meeting of the Transcultural Nursing Society, Flagstaff, AZ.

Welty, T. (1992). Strong heart study finds links between risk factors and CVD in American Indians: CVD rates highest among American Indians in the Northern Plains. In *Fourth National Forum on Cardiovascular Health, Pulmonary Disorders, and Blood Resources* (p. 28). Washington, DC: The National Heart, Lung, and Blood Institute.

Welty, T., Zephier, N., Schweigman, K., Blake, B., & Leonardson, G. (1993). Cancer risk factors in three Sioux Tribes: Use of the Indian-specific health risk appraisal for data collection and analysis. *Alaska Medicine, 35*(4), 265-272.

Wilson, J., Thomann, N., & Gish, C. (1993). *Minority women: Dimensions in health* (U.S. DHHS Region 8 Publication). Greenwood Village, CO: Bachman.

4 Contemporary Research Issues in Hispanic/Latino Women's Health

RUTH E. ZAMBRANA

BRITT K. ELLIS

By the year 2000, Hispanics/Latinos[1] will be the largest minority group in the United States (U.S. Bureau of the Census, 1991). However, little is known about the diverse subgroups that compose this ethnic category. Limited data exist on Hispanic/Latino women and factors that mediate their health status. In general, researchers measure Hispanic/Latino women as a homogeneous category, thus limiting understanding of the unique health needs and health status of subgroup cohorts. The dearth of information on intraethnic differences of Hispanic/Latino women has significantly contributed to a lack of relevant policies and interventions that effectively address their unique issues. If quantitative advances are to be made in comprehending a fuller context of Hispanic/Latino women's health, researchers and other health professionals must initiate

AUTHORS' NOTE: The authors gratefully acknowledge and wish to thank Rosemary Torres, JD, BSN, for her thoughtful review and assistance in the preparation of this chapter, particularly the policy implications for women's health.

42

epidemiologic studies that examine biological, socioeconomic, cultural, behavioral, and other differences among subgroups. The measurement of sociocultural and behavioral risk factors that affect disease patterns, as well as knowledge about the effectiveness of various strategies, are necessary to improve Hispanic/Latino women's health.

The purpose of this chapter is to review and discuss the primary issues central to Hispanic/Latino women's health status in the United States. The chapter provides an overview of Hispanic/Latino health status with a specific focus on Hispanic women. The review is neither comprehensive nor inclusive of all biomedical or behavioral science research in any particular area. The aim is to highlight areas of need. Due to the limited information about Hispanic/Latino health and particularly women's health, as well as the limited data by subgroup, the authors present data on Hispanic men and women. Data on patterns of morbidity and mortality of Hispanic/Latino women, including infectious and noninfectious diseases, the role of acculturation on risk factors and lifestyle behaviors, maternal child health status, and mental health issues, are presented. Data are drawn from published national and state databases and empirical studies. This chapter is designed to provide health and human service professionals with relevant information regarding Hispanic/Latino women's health and to provide researchers with some important research questions and policy recommendations regarding an effective agenda for Hispanic/Latino women's health.

Sociodemographic Profile of Hispanic/Latino Women

The profile of the Hispanic/Latino community is an important key to understanding the community, family, and socioeconomic position of this ethnic group, and it also serves to highlight intragroup differences. Thus data is presented on family structure, poverty rates, and employment and occupational status for each subgroup.

The Hispanic/Latino population is currently composed of 61.2% Mexican (includes Mexican, Mexican American, Chicano), 12% Puerto Rican, 4.8% Cuban, 11% Central and South American, and 11% other Latino (those whose reported origin was Spain, or Latino persons identifying themselves generally as Hispanic, Spanish, Spanish-American, Hispano, Latino). The geographic distribution of Hispanic subpopulations varies considerably by region, with Mexican Americans living primarily throughout the U.S. Southwest, West, and Midwest, Puerto Ricans occupying the Northeast, and Cubans living through-out the Southeast. Although this understanding of geographical placement has aided researchers in targeting and assessing the health status of the aforementioned Hispanic/Latino subgroups, those most often delineated by the category *Central and South American* represent the fastest-growing Hispanic group in the United States. These Latinos have migrated to various areas throughout the United States, but they are found predominantly in Los Angeles and Washington, D.C. Little national attention has been given to the significant cultural differences between the Hispanic/Latino subgroups or to how their experiences in the United States and their countries of origin have affected their health status (U.S. Bureau of the Census, 1991). Health status is integrally related to social and economic status, family structure, and quality of life indicators, as measured by physical environment and availability and access to health and human services. For Hispanic/Latino women, these factors represent an important context in which to examine their health status.

Most Latinos (69%) maintain traditional family structures. However, households headed by a female with no male spouse present are six times more likely to be Latino (24%) than non-Hispanic White (4%). House-holds with a male head and no wife present are almost twice as likely to be Latino (7%) as non-Hispanic White (4%). Among the Latino subgroups, Puerto Rican families are the least likely to be maintained by a married couple (52%) and the most likely to be maintained by a woman with no husband present (43%). Latino families (3.80 people) are larger than non-Hispanic White families (3.13 people). Furthermore, 29% of Latino families have five or more members, compared to only 13% of non-Hispanic White families. Among the subgroups, Mexicans have the highest proportion of families with five or more members (34%), followed by Puerto Ricans (20%), Cubans (16%), Central/South Americans (26%), and Other Latinos (19%).

The poverty rate among Hispanic families was 29.3% in 1993. Latino families earned an average of $23,912 in 1992, compared to

$40,420 for non-Hispanic families. Latino females averaged an annual income of $17,124. Although Hispanics constitute 9% of the population, more that one of every six people living in poverty in the United States are of Hispanic origin. In 1990, the median income of Latino families ($23,200), after adjusting for the increase in the cost of living during the period, was almost equal that of non-Hispanic White families ($23,517) in 1982. In actuality, the median family income for Latino families in 1990 was about 64% of the median income of non-Latino families ($36,300). Family incomes varied substantially among Latino subgroups. The median for Puerto Rican families ($18,000) was the lowest, whereas Cuban families ($31,400) almost matched the income of non-Hispanic Whites, and Mexican families ($23,200) fell somewhere in the middle.

Latino families were more likely to live in poverty than non-Hispanic White families. Based on 1990 income figures, 25% of Latino families fell below the poverty level, as compared to 9.5% of non-Hispanic White families. By 1990, 17% of Latino families in poverty were maintained by people who were 65 years old or older, compared to 5.9% of non-Hispanic White families in poverty. Furthermore, 48.3% of Latino families in poverty were maintained by females without a husband present, compared to 31.7% of non-Hispanic White families in poverty. Among Latino family subgroups, Puerto Rican families were the most likely to be in poverty in 1990 (37.5%). This high poverty rate may be related to the high proportion of families maintained by females without a spouse present. In fact, by 1990 approximately two thirds (64.4%) of such families were in poverty.

Latino males (57%) and Latino females (54%) failed to graduate from college more often than non-Hispanic White males and females (32%). The labor force participation for non-Hispanic White women (57%) was higher than for Latino women (51%). Among the subgroups, Central and South Americans reported the highest labor-force participation, followed by Cubans (55%), Mexicans (51%) and Puerto Ricans (42%). This indicates an increase of Latinas in the workforce between 1983 (41%) and 1991. Latinas 25 years and older (31.2%) were also more likely than non-Hispanic White females their age (22.0%) or men to earn below-poverty wages. Among all employed females, the single largest occupational grouping for both Latinas (40%) and non-Hispanic White women (44%) was technical, sales, and administrative support occupations. However, other differences were also noted. About 16% of Latinas were employed in managerial and professional specialty occupations, compared to 28% of non-Hispanic White women. Also, 26% of Hispanic/Latino women were employed in service occupations, compared to 17% of non-Hispanic White women. Finally, about twice as many Latinas (14%) as non-Hispanic women (8%) held positions as operators, fabricators, and laborers.

These socioeconomic, demographic, and familial context variables demonstrate that a significant proportion of the Hispanic population is at risk or vulnerable to poor health outcomes. Low socioeconomic status is integrally related to living in poor environmental conditions, exposure to more chronic life stressors such as financial instability, less likelihood of having health insurance, and limited access to health care services as a result of institutional discrimination or sociocultural, financial, and other barriers (U.S. Office of the Surgeon General, 1993). Equally important, low socioeconomic status places Hispanic/Latinos, especially women, at increased behavioral risk because of their limited education and limited access to health education information due to language, literacy, cultural, and other barriers.

The Relationship of Acculturation to Behavioral Risk Factors

There is limited empirical work regarding risk factors and specific clinical outcomes for the Hispanic population in general. The available studies have been conducted predominantly in the West and Southwest with Mexican Americans, and most of the current data are derived from the 1982-1984 Hispanic-Health and Nutrition Examination Survey (HHANES).[2]

A significant portion of the studies focused attention on the relationship between acculturation and specific health behaviors or clinical outcomes. One consistent finding has been use of the English language as a principal marker of acculturation (Oetting & Beauvais, 1991). Although acculturation and its measurement are still poorly understood, the findings on acculturation and Hispanic\Latino women's health status, especially among the Mexican American population, are of interest and importance. The following provides a summary of relationships found between acculturation and behavioral risk factors, predominantly from the HHANES national data set:

- Acculturation is positively associated with frequency of alcohol consumption and probability of being a drinker among Cuban, Mexican American, and Puerto Rican women (Black & Markides, 1993).
- Low acculturated Latinas were found to be least likely to engage in illegal drug use and sexual activity with multiple partners, and they also perceived themselves to be at low risk for HIV infection (Nyamathi, Bennett, Leake, Lewis, & Flaskerud, 1993).
- Acculturation was found to be a predictor of multiple sex partners in Mexican American, Cuban American, and Puerto Rican women, with higher levels of acculturation being positively related to history of multiple sex partners (Sabogal, Faigeles, & Catania, 1993).
- Low acculturated Hispanic men with secondary female sexual partners were found to have more positive attitudes toward condom use and to carry condoms on their person more often than highly acculturated men (Marin, Tschann, Gomez, & Kegeles, 1993).
- Spanish-speaking women, however, although they were found to have fewer sexual partners, also reported less condom use than did their non-Hispanic White women (Marin, Gomez, & Tschann, 1993).
- For Mexican Americans, increased acculturation has been found to be directly related to the prevalence of cigarette smoking (Coreil, Ray, & Markides, 1991).
- When Hispanic women identify as smokers, those with higher levels of acculturation were found to smoke more in general than did the less acculturated (Marin, Perez-Stable, & Marin, 1989).
- Level of acculturation affects the prevalence and variation of spousal violence. One third of the most recent incidents reported by Mexican American women born in Mexico were described as rape (by the male partner). Spousal violence affected one fifth of the households in the sample and was shown to be higher in U.S.-born Mexican Americans (Sorenson & Telles, 1991).
- A study examining the relationship between acculturation and cardiovascular disease risk in Mexican American women found that those who have higher levels of acculturation had a lower incidence of obesity overall and less central adiposity (Hazuda, Mitchell, Haffner, & Stern, 1991). Highly acculturated Mexican American men in the same study, however, were shown to have higher levels of obesity and more centrally located body fat.

- Preventive health behaviors are negatively associated with increased acculturation. Less acculturated women were less likely to have had an annual Pap smear, and those over 50 reported never having had a mammogram (Elder et al., 1991). Data from the National Health Interview Survey show that women who spoke predominantly Spanish were the least likely to have had a Pap smear within 3 years prior to the time of interview (Harlan, Bernstein, & Kessler, 1991). Less acculturated Mexican American women were also less likely to have been hospitalized (Markides & Lee, 1991).

Current analyses of the empirical data on the relationship of acculturation to behavioral risk factors and disease patterns support conclusions that more recent Hispanic female immigrants were less likely to engage in smoking cigarettes, drinking alcohol, and drug use, when compared to Hispanic/Latino women who were born and raised in the United States or have been in the United States for 10 years or more (Stephen, Foote, Hendershot, & Schoenborn, 1994). These data suggest that exposure to dominant cultural norms in U.S. society contributes to a decrease in traditional norms and values regarding the sociocultural behaviors of Hispanic/Latino women. Thus the literature has defined traditional gender-associated Hispanic/Latino behaviors as protective behaviors. However, this approach assumes that adaptation to a new culture simultaneously and linearly signifies a decrease in identification with the culture of origin.

The assumption of linear acculturation does not examine the multidimensionality of a process of cultural adaptation, and how this process may negatively affect an individual's health status. Thus, the interaction of low socioeconomic status and cultural adaptation needs to be more closely examined. Aside from language acquisition, central variables of interest include country of origin, rural/urban origin, number of years in the United States, level of education, socioeconomic status, access to health services, sociocultural barriers and exposure to institutional discrimination, and situational cultural preferences and attitudes. A multidisciplinary examination, a more precise definition of acculturation, and refined measurement of changes in cultural attitudes and norms regarding health behaviors have great potential for contributing to a better understanding of the differential patterns of mortality and morbidity among Hispanic/Latino women.

Morbidity and Mortality Patterns

The leading causes of death among Latinas are heart diseases, diabetes, and cancer (breast, lung). For example, Mexican-origin females account for 48% of all deaths from cancer in Texas. However, the prevalence and incidence of these diseases vary significantly across Latino subgroups (Desenclos & Hahn, 1992; Frank-Stromberg, 1991; U.S. Department of Health & Human Services [DHHS], 1991). There is a paucity of information on the epidemiology of disease patterns for Hispanic/Latino women and the risk factors that may account for morbidity and mortality patterns (Zambrana, Kelly, & Raskin, 1994). This section reviews the the few existing studies on chronic diseases and risk factors available on the general Hispanic population by subgroup and gender.

Overall, Hispanic/Latino groups are at a markedly increased risk for diabetes mellitus type II, gallbladder disease, hypertension, stroke, hypercholesterolemia, cardiovascular disease (CVD) mortality, and obesity. Hispanics have also been found to have lower CVD knowledge levels when compared to their non-Hispanic White counterparts (Ford & Jones, 1991). Although the research regarding CVD is inconclusive, some studies have examined the increased mortality rates following myocardial infarction in Hispanic/Latino women. In a study of Mexican American women in Texas, it was found that Latinos experienced a 37% greater 28-day mortality rate than their non-Hispanic White female counterparts (Goff et al., 1993). Interestingly, the cardiovascular risk profile for U.S.-born Mexican Americans was more favorable than the profile for their Mexican-born counterparts (Mitchell, Stern, Haffner, Hazuda, & Patterson, 1990). Hyperinsulinemia, also prevalent in Mexican Americans, has been associated with obesity, elevated triglyceride levels, low levels of high-density lipoprotein cholesterol (HDL), and hypertension. Results from the San Antonio Heart Study indicate that high levels of fasting insulin were more strongly correlated with a decrease in HDL in Hispanic/Latino women (Mitchell, Haffner, Hazuda, Valdez, & Stern, 1992). Thus, Latinas, compared to their male counterparts and non-Hispanic White males and females, experienced greater incidence of CVD risk in relation to the protective factors of HDL, as affected by higher insulin levels.

Diabetes disproportionately affects the Hispanic population, although there are different patterns by subgroup. Diabetes has been diagnosed in 24% of Mexican Americans, 26% of Puerto Ricans, and 16% of Cuban Americans (Flegal et al., 1991). Diabetic Mexican American women have been found to have lower levels of education and employment than their non-diabetic counterparts. They have also been found to have higher prevalence of kidney problems, hypertension, and cataracts. The duration of diabetes was also related to stroke and activity limitation in both women and men (Zhang, Markides, & Lee, 1991). Gestational diabetes mellitus (GDM) is the most common pregnancy-related problem among Mexican American women, occurring at three times the rate experienced by non-Hispanic women. Mexican American women with GDM were more likely to have larger and longer babies, and obese mothers were more likely to have cesarean sections and preterm labor. The infants of Mexican-American obese mothers with GDM had higher rates of polycythemia and sepsis (Hollingsworth, Vaucher, & Yamamoto, 1991).

Mexican American diabetic women have also been found to be at increased risk for gallbladder disease (Haffner, Diehl, Mitchell, Stern, & Hazuda, 1990). Risk factors for gallstone disease in Mexican American women were age, menopause, body mass index, sum of four skinfolds, diabetes, impaired glucose tolerance, and use of oral contraceptives (Maurer, Everhart, Knowler, Shawker, & Roth, 1990). The prevalence of gallstone disease for Mexican American women was 1.5 times that of Cuban women and 1.7 times that of Puerto Rican women, reaching 44.1% among Mexican American women of 60 to 74 years of age (Maurer et al., 1989).

Although many types of cancer appear to affect Hispanics at lower rates than their non-Hispanic White counterparts, some forms of cancer have a higher incidence in Hispanic/Latino women. The rate of cancer of the cervix among Latinas living in New York City was 2.5 times higher than the rate among non-Hispanic White women (Wolfgang, Semeiks, & Burnett, 1991). Hispanic/Latino women, particularly Puerto Rican women, have been found to have Pap smears and mammograms at lower rates than their African American and non-Hispanic White counterparts. Latinas who report a perception that health outcomes are more controlled by medical professionals are less likely to engage in preventive behaviors, such as breast self-examination (Bundek, Marks, & Richardson, 1993). There is limited data on the risk factors that may account for these disease patterns. However, access to and use of appropriate services may be affected by sociocultural barriers such as attitudes and beliefs; English-language proficiency and literacy; and financial barriers such as lack of child care, transportation, and the need to meet immediate needs (as opposed to those of a long-term nature).

Infectious Diseases

The prevalence rates of many infectious diseases are much greater among Hispanic/Latino women than among non-Hispanic White women. Although Latinas represent approximately 9% of the U.S. female population, they account for 21% of AIDS cases among women (Centers for Disease Control, 1993.) HIV infection and AIDS are especially prevalent among Puerto Rican women living in the Northeast. Research has shown that Puerto Rican women living in New York City are at higher risk of having AIDS than any other racial or ethnic group, including African American women (Menendez, 1990). Factors in this community that contribute to increased risk are intravenous drug use, patterns in migration and marriage, and socioeconomic status. Little research has been done to evaluate the incidence of HIV and AIDS among other groups of Hispanic/Latino women. HIV infection transmission factors and incidence of HIV and AIDS-related conditions should be examined urgently among recently immigrated Latinas from Central and South America and the Dominican Republic.

Female physiology has been shown to place women at 20 times greater risk of infection through vaginal-penis sex with an infected male. Thus, women are more vulnerable to infection if condoms are not used at the time of intercourse. Research has shown that heterosexual Hispanic males often do not perceive themselves to be at risk, even if they are engaging in unprotected intercourse (Vega, Kolody, Hwang, & Noble, 1993). According to the National AIDS Behavioral Surveys, 17% of Hispanic males living in high-risk cities reported having had multiple partners. In another study, it was found that among Hispanics with secondary partners, only 29% used condoms on a

regular basis (Sabogal et al., 1993). Local surveys of Latino males in
New York City found that approximately one third engaged in unprotected sex with a secondary partner. Predictors of multiple sexual
partners among Hispanic/Latino women were marital status, age,
Hispanic subgroup, and level of acculturation. The incidence of unprotected sex with secondary partners among Hispanic males, combined with a low perceived risk of HIV infection, places Hispanic/
Latino women at an ever-increasing risk for HIV transmission through
vaginal sex.

There are multiple scientific and ethical reasons that justify immediate and increased concern for the welfare of Hispanic/Latino
women in relation to HIV and AIDS. Comparison of the results of
AIDS-related surveys conducted in 1988 and 1990 by the National
Center for Health Statistics demonstrated that HIV/AIDS-related
knowledge among Hispanic/Latino women in Los Angeles did not
improve between 1988 and 1990 (Flaskerud & Uman, 1993). Targeted
programs to educate Latinas have been few, often ineffective, and
poorly evaluated. Many of these programs have not been specifically
designed to take into account cultural, language, and educational
context. Low-income Hispanic/Latino communities are experiencing disproportionate amounts of HIV infection through heterosexual
transmission. Data relating to the transmission and prevalence of
sexually transmitted diseases (STDs) among women are often poorly
collected and sparse. In fact, syphilis and gonorrhea are the only two
STDs that are mandatorily reported; thus, information is unavailable
for other STDs, which tend to infect women at higher rates and to be
more problematic in their treatment and cure. A serious consequence
of STDs is that they lower immunological protection and increase the
chances of HIV infection during unprotected sexual activity.

There is a critical need for data relating to the incidence of
human papilloma virus (HPV), herpes, pelvic inflammatory disease,
and chlamydia among women in general, and specifically among
Hispanic/Latino female subpopulations. Research has indicated that
herpes simplex virus II is strongly associated with female gender,
Hispanic ethnicity, number of sexual partners, limited level of education, and older age. Foreign-born Hispanics were found to have a
greater incidence than those born within the United States (Siegel
et al., 1992). African American and Hispanic communities in New

York City have been found to have disproportionate levels of early latent and congenital syphilis (Ong, Rubin, Brome-Bunting, & Labes, 1991). Hispanic ethnicity has been shown to be a factor in the screening for STDs among women. According to the 1988 National Survey of Family Growth, only 27% of Hispanic/Latino women had been tested the year prior to the survey, compared with 47% of African American females (Mosher & Aral, 1991).

Recently, specific strains of HPV have been linked to the incidence of cervical cancer among women. The lack of data, combined with the fact that Latinas are least likely to have received a Pap smear within the past 1 to 3 years, makes it imperative to conduct studies to determine the prevalence of strain-specific HPV among Latinas and to identify barriers to treatment and screening. The high incidence of STDs among Latinas exacerbates the risk of HIV infection and contributes to a host of treatment and reproductive problems among this population. Urgent education, research, screening, and treatment programs are needed to curb the prevalence of STDs, STD-specific transmission factors, and related behaviors among subgroups of Latinas.

Other infectious diseases that are currently prevalent in the Hispanic community are hepatitis B and tuberculosis. Although hepatitis B has not been found to be prevalent among rural Mexican American women, rates of infection in pregnant Latinas of Caribbean and Latin American origin have been documented (Dinsmoor & Gibbs, 1990). In addition, Isoniazid-induced hepatitis among pregnant and postpartum Hispanics has been found among Latinas attending county health prenatal clinics. The use of Isoniazid to treat those with tuberculosis is prevalent throughout immigrant communities. The authors found that Latinas in prenatal care clinics had 2.5 times the risk of incurring Isoniazid hepatitis B and four times the mortality rate, when compared to previously collected data from the Public Health Service (Franks, Binkin, Snider, Rokaw, & Becker, 1989). Recent data show an increase in rates of tuberculosis, especially among Hispanic immigrant women (Rassin et al., 1993).

The spread of infectious diseases is integrally related to environmental conditions, access to preventive and primary health care services, socioeconomic factors, and health behaviors, which are strongly influenced by levels of education and access to information. For a significant number of Hispanic/Latino women, such nonmedical factors are central in understanding their increased risk for disease. Infectious diseases such as HIV/AIDS, STDs, and tuberculosis represent serious medical risk conditions for pregnant Hispanic/Latino women and their offspring.

Maternal and Child Health: Outcomes and Practices

Overall, Hispanic/Latino women have higher fertility rates and tend to begin childbearing at younger ages. They are also less likely to use health services, to have public or private insurance, and to have access to prenatal and postnatal services. In 1987, the percentages of women receiving late (not until the third trimester) or no prenatal care at all were 12.7% and 11.1% for Latinas and African American women respectively, compared with 5% for non-Hispanic women (DHHS, 1991).

Patterns of use of prenatal care vary by Hispanic subgroup. Puerto Rican women are the most likely to receive late or no prenatal care (17%), followed by Central American (13.5%) and Mexican-origin (13%) women (DHHS, 1991). Several studies have demonstrated that Mexican-born women were the least likely of all groups in California to begin prenatal care during the first trimester. Among Mexican-origin women, Mexican-born women were less likely to initiate care in the first trimester than either African American or Mexican American women (Zambrana, Dunkel-Schetter, & Scrimshaw, 1991). Mexican immigrant women confront a number of barriers to prenatal care: low income; low education; limited financial access to prenatal care programs, including pregnancy-related social services; monolingual Spanish speaking; stress of being immigrant; and possible stress of being undocumented.

However, despite the low initiation rates of prenatal care in the first trimester by Latino women, this group has rates of low birth weight (LBW) comparable to non-Hispanic White women. In 1987, the LBW rates among Mexican, Cuban, and Central and South American infants ranged from 5.7% to 5.9% per 1000 compared to 5.6% for non-Hispanic White women. The LBW rate among Puerto Rican infants was

9.3% (Duany & Pittman, 1990). Although they are at relatively low risk of LBW, Latino infants are at greater risk of being born prematurely. In 1987, the preterm rates (infants born at less than 37 weeks completed gestation) were 9% for Cuban women, 12.6% for Puerto Rican women, and 11% for Mexican-origin women, compared to 8.5% for non-Hispanic White women.

Several studies have found that generational status (or nativity) of the mother is an important predictor of LBW (Guendelman, Gould, Hudes, & Eskenazi, 1990; Scribner & Dwyer, 1989). U.S.-born (second-generation) Mexican women were more likely than Mexican-born women to give birth to infants under 2,500 grams. This occurred despite the fact that, compared to Mexican-born women, U.S.-born women had more education, better incomes, and higher health care use rates (Guendelman et al., 1990). However, when we examine birth outcomes among Hispanic subgroups, the data show that Puerto Rican women have similar birth outcomes to African American women (DHHS, 1991). Research also suggests that the association of maternal LBW to infant LBW appears to be stronger in Latinas than in non-Hispanic White and African American women (Leff et al., 1992). Furthermore, it appears that country of origin and time within the United States seem to also negatively affect birth outcome. In summary, there is evidence to suggest that Latinas born in the United States and those that immigrated early in their childhood have increased behavioral risk factors related to unfavorable birth outcome. Although the factors that may account for this outcome are poorly understood in the research community, preliminary findings suggest that the exposure of late immigration to the United States may in fact increase the probability of a Latino woman having a social support network, as well as the assistance of her male partner.

Acculturation has also been shown to affect the initiation of breast feeding in Mexican American mothers. Mothers who reported lower levels of acculturation were more likely to initiate breast feeding than were women who showed higher levels of acculturation. Infant-feeding practices of Latino mothers may also have a detrimental affect on infant health. Mexican and Central American women have been found to introduce solid foods and inappropriate liquids at premature ages. These practices can lead to allergies, dysentery, increased rate of infection, and choking. Latina mothers have also been found to prop baby bottles because of feeding-time constraints, thus placing the infant at risk of choking (Ellis, Feldman, Anliker, & Bernstein, 1994). Breast feeding is vital for both the health of the infant and the bonding process of mother to child, which suggests that breast feeding and infant-feeding education among more acculturated Latinas is warranted.

Psychosocial Health and Mental Well-Being of Hispanic/Latino Women

The relationship between health and mental health status or psychosocial functioning has become a focal area of inquiry in recent years. Chronic life stressors and social supports from family, friends, and institutions are increasingly heralded as important mediators in understanding the links between individual and group vulnerability, health status, and clinical outcome, particularly in low-income Hispanic/Latino women and other women of color (Lillie-Blanton, Martinez, Taylor, & Robinson, 1993).

Analysis of the role acculturation plays in mental health status among the Mexican American population demonstrates that as people begin to advance socially and economically in U.S. society, they often lose traditional resources and ethnically based social support networks, contributing to increased levels of distress. This distress seems to abate as people grow older and reformulate links between themselves and their native culture (Kaplan & Marks, 1990). Birthplace also appears to affect mental health status among Mexican Americans. Those born in the United States were found to have higher levels of depression, compared to their Mexican-born counterparts (Golding & Burnam, 1990; Moscicki, Locke, Rae, & Boyd, 1989). In addition, being female and having low socioeconomic status also predisposed Mexican Americans to depressive symptomatology (Moscicki et al., 1989). Low acculturation has also been shown to have a negative affect on mental health status among Mexican American women and older adults (Garcia & Marks, 1989).

Many areas of psychosocial functioning require inquiry. The relationship of mental functioning and changes in family structure demands attention, as Latino/Hispanic family structures change.

The long-standing support of extended family may be weakening as a result of high mobility and the varied living arrangements used by immigrants in large urban areas. The sense of loss experienced by recent immigrants may contribute to increased depression. In a study examining the use of pediatric emergency services with a sample of Mexican and Central American immigrants in Los Angeles, the data showed that the women reported high levels of mental distress and low levels of ability to cope. These data suggest women's health status may contribute to a delay in health care for the child (Zambrana, Ell, Dorrington, Wachsman, & Hodge, 1994). The particular situation of Central American refugees must be examined within the political context in their country of origin. Over half of a recent sample of Central American immigrants who had immigrated as a result of war and political strife demonstrated symptomology consistent with a diagnosis of posttraumatic stress disorder (PTSD).

A focus on the affect of PTSD on the physical and psychosocial health of Central and South American women in relation to the acculturation process is an important area of investigation (Cervantes, Salgado de Snyder, & Padilla, 1989; Dorrington, 1995). There has been no known national effort to determine the incidence and effects of PTSD among Central and South Americans in general, especially research on how the disorder may affect the lives of women and their families. In addition, the instrumentation needed to measure PTSD must be formulated and adapted to accurately measure this variable and its affect on the health status of Hispanic/Latino women. A focus on co-morbid conditions such as alcoholism and chemical use and dependency should be examined with groups experiencing PTSD. The set of relationships among physical or functional status, mental health status, and perceived health status require systematic investigation among Hispanic/Latino women, with attention to differences by place of birth, Hispanic subgroup, and age.

Research and Policy Implications
of Women's Health for Hispanic/Latino Women

Women's health research has captured the attention of a significant portion of the American public and, in some circles, it is seen as an issue whose time has come. Extensive and high-profile media coverage of women's health topics has increased awareness of factors influencing the health status of women of diverse national origins. Published findings of studies examining scientific questions regarding women's health issues in multidisciplinary professional journals such as the *Journal of the American Medical Women's Association*, the *Journal of Women's Health*, and the *Journal of the American Public Health Association* support the conclusion, by some, that women's health is experiencing a period of enlightened thinking (National Institutes of Health, 1992).

The dearth of research data on Hispanic/Latino women has been repeatedly documented by multidisciplinary Hispanic/Latino scientists. Currently, researchers are making important contributions in efforts to close the knowledge gaps and to educate the scientific communities and policymakers regarding the multiple health needs of Hispanic/Latino women during all stages of their lives. For example, the landmark 1992-1993 Hispanic/Latino Health Initiative, spearheaded by former U.S. Surgeon General Antonia C. Novello, MD, included specific recommendations to improve Hispanic/Latino health. The seminal 1993 report, *One Voice, One Vision*, reflects the longstanding diligence and commitment on the part of the Hispanic/ Latino community to provide vision and leadership in addressing socioeconomic, environmental, biological, and other factors established as detrimental to the physical and mental health of female members of Hispanic/Latino families in the United States.

Research agendas on specific focal areas for Hispanic/Latino women have been emerging over the last decade. The review of literature in this chapter reflects a historical underrepresentation of this group of women in scientific investigations. The contemporary inventory of available data too often only describes selected disease patterns for Hispanic/Latino women, predominantly Mexican American women, without a context for understanding the multiple factors that influence these health outcomes. Thus, a paradigm for understanding the health status of Hispanic/Latino women must be embedded in a sociodemographic, psychosocial, and sociocultural context to significantly advance knowledge in women's health (Zambrana, 1994). There are multiple areas in which research efforts must be undertaken if scientific knowledge gaps are to be remedied. Morbidity and mortality rates can serve as guides for future research investigations. Studies on heart disease, hypertension, infectious disease, and specific cancers in subgroups of Hispanic/Latino women are warranted. For example, the examination of the relationship among multiple roles and their perceived burden, psychosocial stressors (including chronic life events), and perceived institutional discrimination in Hispanic/Latino women with coronary heart disease and hypertension is one of many important questions.

Diabetes is a prevalent chronic condition among Hispanic/Latino women. The role of chronic life stressors, nutritional patterns, and possibly genetic vulnerability also merit immediate and systematic investigation. Intragroup differences between Mexican American, Puerto Rican, and Cuban women in different geographical locations, controlling for socioeconomic status, may provide useful information on patterns that may account for intragroup differences in treatment effectiveness among these groups. A second important area is STDs. Current data suggest that multiple partners, traditional cultural norms and practices, and limited access to preventive and primary care services are contributing to the significant number of Hispanic/Latino women with STDs. The research in this area should focus on examining cultural attitudes and norms among both Hispanic men and women to determine the factors that contribute to the sexual transmission of infectious diseases, and then examine these patterns within geographic regions, by Hispanic subgroup. STDs have serious implications, such as infertility and increased risk of HIV infection.

Data on pregnancy outcome have received some attention in the last decade. However, the studies have not fully identified nor examined the protective factors or behaviors that contribute to improved outcome, nor has adequate research been conducted to determine how those factors may change for Hispanic/Latino women who are born in the United States or have resided here for long periods of time. Puerto Rican women, who have the least favorable birth outcomes, have received the least attention. Intragroup studies are required that examine the role of factors such as health behaviors, nutritional patterns, and maternal attitudes on pregnancy outcome, and how these factors change with greater length of time in the United States and for U.S.-born Hispanics. In other words, research should begin to identify the processes that sustain culturally protective factors, and those processes that may contribute to culturally decreasing protective factors. Future investigations in this area should be guided by a more multidimensional model that examines the relationships among ethnic identity, socioeconomic status, behavioral risk factors, psychosocial factors (including violence in the home and community), and birth outcomes. Several studies have suggested relationships between violence, substance use, and pregnancy (Amaro, 1993). The data suggest that the study of pregnancy for Latino women must be studied within a social, cultural, and community context.

Cancer research has received noticeably limited attention in Latino groups, due to a lower incidence of the disease than non-Hispanic Whites experience. However, Hispanic/Latino women are displaying increasing rates of breast, cervix, and colon cancers. The incidence and prevalence of these cancers vary by geographic region. To ensure an informed and timely set of investigations, surveillance mechanisms are needed to monitor increases in cancer rates in Latinos, and cancer patterns must be examined by country of origin (Valdez, Delgado, Cervantes, & Bowler, 1993). In addition, the relationships between STDs and cervical cancer, and cancers in later adulthood and old age require scrutiny.

The research agenda for Hispanic/Latino women must be guided by an informed multidimensional paradigm. The study of disease patterns and the eventual individual health status of Hispanic/ Latino women is influenced by multiple factors, biomedical data, health behaviors, nutritional patterns, sociocultural barriers, and institutional access. The importance of expanding our lens to better understand how socioeconomic status, ethnicity, Hispanic gender, and health status interact can no longer be ignored.

Policy Implications: Barriers to Hispanic/Latino Women's Research

The research agenda for Hispanic/Latino women has been articulated, and their underrepresentation in scientific investigations has also been confirmed. At present, initiatives to address the health of Latino populations, especially women, have not translated into easily discernible and effective policy or allocation of sufficient resources. However, recent policy initiatives focused on women's health have established the scientific rationale for substantially increasing the participation of Latino/Hispanic women in future investigations.

An important milestone in women's health research occurred in 1983, when the Assistant Secretary for Health established a U.S. Public Health Service Task Force on Women's Health Issues. The task force report (U.S. Public Health Service, 1985) presented "discussions of a broad array of women's health issues across the life stages and particularly in the context of the sociological changes in the United States in the latter years of the 20th century." One of the most important recommendations emanating from the Task Force Report was, "Biomedical and behavioral research should be expanded to ensure emphasis on conditions and diseases unique to, or more prevalent in, women of all age groups" (Kirschstein, 1991, pp. 291-293). Subsequently, the Congressional Caucus on Women's Issues responded to the groundswell of interest in women's issues and stimulated federal offices and agencies within the U.S. Public Health Service to meaningfully address women's health needs. At the request of the caucus, the General Accounting Office initiated an investigation that determined that women of diverse racial and ethnic origins were disproportionately excluded from participation in human research studies funded by the National Institutes of Health (NIH). In response to this finding, NIH established the Office of Research on Women's Health in 1990, to develop a research agenda for women's health, ensuring greater inclusion of all women in clinical studies and increasing opportunities for women in biomedical careers (NIH, 1992).

An important outcome of these policy initiatives was a set of provisions, stipulated in the law, that specifically addresses the inclusion of women and minorities in clinical studies. These areas include whether the participation of women and minorities is judged appropriate with respect to the health of the subjects and the purpose of the research, or inappropriate under such other circumstances as the Director of NIH may designate. The policy requires that, in addition to the continuing inclusion of women and members of minority groups in all NIH-supported biomedical and behavioral research involving human subjects, women and members of minorities and their subpopulations must be included in all research on human subjects. Furthermore, it is stipulated that for Phase III clinical trials, women and minorities and their subpopulations must be included to assure that valid analyses of differences in intervention effect can be accomplished; that cost is not an acceptable reason for excluding these groups; and that programs and support for outreach efforts to recruit these groups into clinical studies should be initiated.

Scientific, legal, social, and ethical issues related to the inclusion of women in human-subject research were recently revisited by Congress. The NIH Revitalization Act of 1993, signed by President Bill Clinton on June 10, 1993, mandates a number of actions to further ensure diverse representation of women and minorities in publicly funded health studies. According to PL 103-43, the NIH is required to revise existing guidelines governing the inclusion of women and minorities in studies involving human-subject research.[3] These guidelines are science-driven and represent the opportunity to foster collaboration between stakeholders in the human research enterprise. The goal of these initiatives is to determine whether the intervention or therapy being studied has different effects on women or men or members of minority groups and their subpopulations. Of crucial importance, inclusion of racial and ethnic populations by subgroup and gender permits researchers to collect data on subpopulations where knowledge gaps exist.[4]

The nature of this mandate was compellingly described in the two-volume 1994 Institute of Medicine report on *Women and Health Research*. The report includes scientific suggestions for assessment of survey instruments, recruitment procedures, and other methodologies used in the majority or other population(s), with the objective of determining their feasibility, applicability, validity, and cultural competence/relevance to a particular minority group or subpopulation.

Concern remains about whether leadership in addressing the concerns of Hispanic/Latino women will emerge from any of the new alliances and partnerships among stakeholders, such as Hispanic/Latino study participants and researchers, federal agencies responsible for addressing the health needs of Hispanic/Latino women, and representatives of the private-sector research industry, such as pharmaceutical companies and foundations. A. C. Novello, the former U.S. Surgeon General, discussed the challenges that the American health care system confronts in developing "the requisite empirical base and community representation to ensure that this process adaptation and expanded provision will be coherent, efficacious, and humane" (Novello, Wise, & Kleinman, 1991, p. 253). Perhaps part of the answer lies in determining the extent to which opportunities present during this period of "enlightened thinking" regarding women and minority health will be accessible to and used by Hispanic/ Latino public policy and scientific researchers. Traditionally, the ability of administrators of the federal, state, and county health departments to effectively address health issues of Hispanic/Latino women has been severely constrained. Multiple barriers have been identified as contributing to the continued existence of gaps in knowledge. These factors include inadequate data collection systems, lack of funding to collect additional data, lack of representation of Hispanic administrators, and lack of a political voice to present the needs of this group (Furino, 1991, pp. 255-257; U.S. Office of the Surgeon General, 1993).

Thus, minority—particularly multidisciplinary Hispanic/Latino— investigators, clinicians, ethicists, attorneys, and other health experts must assume a more proactive role in designing and conducting biomedical and social research so that it will benefit both the scientific community and under-served groups in our society. Although this mandate parts from traditional research approaches, strategies have been developed to assure that research becomes a critical tool in the advancement of knowledge for the collective good.

Research Strategies for Enhancing Participation of Hispanic/Latino Women

Recommendations for solving complex problems affecting participation in research studies have come from many sources, including Hispanic community leaders, multidisciplinary investigators, administrators, and scientists at leading research institutions across the country. Important perspectives and recommendations regarding strategies for increasing the reliability, validity, and legitimacy of research in Hispanic communities have been proposed. There is a general consensus among Hispanic academic and policy scientists that the principles of inclusion should mean involving representatives of the study populations in planning the study so as to ensure mutually acceptable decision making. The development of knowledge of our diverse communities must involve effective partnerships among communities, their representatives, and research centers. For example, culturally sensitive/bilingual outreach workers should work with appropriate community groups (for example, churches, social service agencies, community-based organizations, and local businesses) to discuss potential studies and identify and recruit study subjects. Second, the study design and procedures must be linguistically and culturally appropriate, taking into account the literacy level of the particular Hispanic subgroups involved. The Hispanic subgroups must be identified with specific ethnic, racial, and socioeconomic indicators. The research team must also include Hispanics at both junior- and senior-level positions who are familiar and knowledgable in substantive and methodological areas and characteristics of the target population. The goal is to train new Hispanic investigators and to increase their career opportunities in research.

Third, investigators must, in principle, include research subjects as full partners in the research effort. To this end the researchers should assume the following responsibilities:

> ensure that study subjects understand the purpose of the study and understand the benefit to them personally and to their community;
>
> recruit the family, not just the individual, to participate;
>
> build on the stronger concern that many of these subjects have for their children's health rather than their own. If their children are enrolled in a study, they may be more likely to become involved.

In addition, strategies must be formulated to help subjects develop a pride of ownership in the study and to ensure that study personnel who work with subjects are bicultural/bilingual and sensitive to subjects' concerns and fears. A mutual relationship of trust, respect, and honesty is crucial. Study participation and cooperation can be enhanced by the following:

> ensuring that the subjects' sense of their importance to the study and their personal worth is continually reinforced;

providing transportation, child care, and expanded, flexible scheduling of visits to research sites; and

reimbursing subjects (providing financial incentives) for participation.[5]

Last, the purpose of clinical research must include a benefit to the participants that is integral to the ethical responsibility of the investigators. Thus investigators must provide follow-up to participants and their community once the study is completed, by sharing results and benefits. Specifically, investigators can provide technical assistance to a local community-based organization to secure funds for a program that builds on knowledge gained from the study.

Clearly, the necessity, challenges, and opportunities to contribute significantly to Hispanic/Latino women's health research have been articulated. The complexity and multiple needs of the Hispanic/Latino community require focused attention and increased allocation of resources. As a result of recent legislative and policy developments, individuals of both genders and all racial and ethnic origins will be more actively recruited for inclusion in human subject research. Minority institutions, physicians, and researchers will be approached to participate in clinical studies, and they should also be prepared to become leading investigators or participants in research to be funded by NIH, other federal and state agencies, and foundations. Scientific, legal, ethical, and social principles must guide inquiry, remedy, and justice. Where Hispano/Latino health is concerned—it truly is time for data, time for action.

Notes

1. Hispanic/Latino women will be used to refer to women from Mexico, Puerto Rico, Cuba, and Central America. The designation *Hispanic* is a federal designation used in national and state reporting systems. *Latino* is a self-designated term by members of different groups. These terms will be used together or separately without preference or prejudice.

2. The HHANES represents the first national effort to collect and analyze data by Hispanic subgroup. Although these data were collected 10 years ago, they represent the only baseline data available for the Hispanic population. A second national survey of HHANES is currently being implemented, using a sample of only Mexican-origin population. The decision to include only one group represents a major setback in terms of the importance of collecting national epidemiologic data over time. Further, it

excludes the Puerto Rican group, which consistently demonstrates the least favorable health outcomes.

3. Thus, proposed guidelines which were published in the March 18, 1994, issue of the *Federal Register* "supersede and strengthen the previous policies, NH/ADAMHA Policy Concerning the Inclusion of Women in Study Populations and ADAMHA/NH Policy Concerning the Inclusion of Minorities in Studies Populations, published in the NH GUIDE FOR GRANTS AND CONTRACTS, 1990." The revised NH inclusion guidelines apply to applications for fiscal year 1995 funding (*Federal Register*, Vol. 59. No. 59. Monday, March 28, 1994. 14508-14513.)

4. The Director of the NIH shall ensure that women and members of minority groups and their subpopulations are included as subjects in biomedical and behavioral research studies funded by NIH. The NIH Director, in consultation with the Directors of the Office of Research on Women's Health and the Office of Research on Minority Health, shall conduct or support outreach programs for the recruitment of women and members of minority groups as subjects in the projects of clinical (human subject) research. The Director of NIH is charged with the responsibility for ensuring that every trial receiving NIH support "is designed and carried out in a manner sufficient to provide for a valid analysis of whether the variables being studied in the trial affect women or members of minority groups differently than other subjects in the trial." Of particular importance is a provision of the law that does not allow costs to be considered in determining whether such inclusion is inappropriate. Exclusion is allowable, however, if there is substantial scientific difference in variables between women and men, or minority groups.

5. These suggestions are summarized from the Public Hearing of Hispanic/Latino scientists, who provided public testimony to NIH on March 29-30, 1993. A significant number of these recommendations are also incorporated into Institute of Medicine, 1994.

References

Amaro, H. (1993, July 19-21). *Using national health data systems to inform Hispanic women's health.* Paper presented at the National Center for Health Statistics, Public Health Conference on Records and Statistics. Washington, DC.

Black, S. A., & Markides, K. S. (1993). Acculturation and alcohol consumption in Puerto Rican, Cuban-American, and Mexican-American women in the United States. *American Journal of Public Health, 83*(6), 890-893.

Bundek, N. I., Marks, G., & Richardson, J. L. (1993). Role of health locus of control beliefs in cancer screening of elderly Hispanic women. *Health Psychology, 12*(3), 193-199.

Centers for Disease Control. (1993, January 7). Advance report of final mortality statistics, 1990. *Morbidity and Mortality Weekly Report, 41,* 7.

Cervantes, R. C., Salgado de Snyder, V. N., & Padilla, A. M. (1989). Posttraumatic stress in immigrants from Central American and Mexico. *Hospital and Community Psychiatry, 40*(6), 615-619.

Coreil, J., Ray, L. A., & Markides, K. S. (1991). Predictors of smoking among Mexican-Americans: Findings from the Hispanic HANES. *Preventive Medicine, 30*(4), 508-517.

Desenclos, J. A., & Hahn, R. A. (1992, November 6). Years of potential life lost before age 65, by race, Hispanic origin, and sex—United States, 1986-1988. *Morbidity and Mortality Weekly Report, 42*.

Dinsmoor, M. J., & Gibbs, R. S. (1990). Prevalence of asymptomatic hepatitis B infection in pregnant Mexican American women. *Obstetrics and Gynecology, 766*(2), 239-240.

Dorrington, C. (1995). Central American refugees in Los Angeles: Adjustment of children and families. In R. E. Zambrana (Ed.), *Understanding Latino families: Scholarship, policy, and practice* (pp. 107-129) Thousand Oaks, CA: Sage.

Duany, L., & Pittman, K. (1990). *Latino youths at a crossroads*. Washington, DC: Children's Defense Fund.

Elder, J. P., Castro, F. G., de Moor, C., Mayer, J., Candelaria, J. I., Campbell, N., Talavera G., & Ware, L. M. (1991). Differences in cancer-risk-related behaviors in Latino and non-Hispanic adults. *Preventive Medicine, 20*(6), 751-763.

Ellis, B. K., Feldman, R., Anliker, J. A., & Bernstein, P. (1994, October 30-November 3). *Infant feeding practices of Central and South American women*. Paper presented at the American Public Health Association, 122nd annual meeting, Washington, DC.

Flaskerud, J. H., & Uman, G. (1993). Directions for AIDS education for Hispanic women based on analyses of survey findings. *Public Health Reports, 108*(3), 298-304.

Flegal, K. M., Ezzati, T. M., Harris, M. I., Haynes, S. G., Juarez, R. Z., Knowler, W. C., Perez-Stable, E. J., & Stern, M. P. (1991). Prevalence of diabetes in Mexican Americans, Cubans, and Puerto Ricans from the Hispanic Health and Nutrition Examination Survey, 1982-1984. *Diabetes Care, 14*(7), 628-638.

Ford, E. S., & Jones, D. H. (1991). Cardiovascular health knowledge in the United States: Findings from the National Health Interview Survey, 1988. *Preventive Medicine, 20*(6), 725-736.

Franks, A. L., Binkin, N. J., Snider, D. E., Jr., Rokaw, W. M., & Becker, S. (1989). Isoniazid hepatitis among pregnant and postpartum Hispanic patients. *Public Health Reports, 104*(2), 151-155.

Frank-Stromberg, M. (1991). Changing demographics in the United States. *Cancer, 67*, 772-778.

Furino A. (1991). Health status among Hispanics: Major themes and new priorities. *Journal of the American Medical Association, 265*, 255-257.

Garcia, M., & Marks, G. (1989). Depressive symptomatology among Mexican American adults: An examination with the CES-D scale. *Psychiatry Research, 27*(2), 137-148.

Goff, D. C., Jr., Varas, C., Ramsey, D. J., Wear, M. L., Labarthe, D. R., & Nichaman, M. Z. (1993). Mortality after hospitalization for myocardial infarction among Mexican Americans and non-Hispanic Whites: The Corpus Christi Heart Project. *Ethnicity and Disease, 3*(1), 55-63.

Golding, J. M., & Burnam, M. A. (1990). Immigration, stress, and depressive symptoms in a Mexican-American community. *Journal of Mental and Nervous Disorders, 178*(3), 161-171.

Guendelman, S., Gould, J. B., Hudes, M., & Eskenazi, B. (1990). Generational diffferences in perinatal health among the Mexican American population: Findings from HHANES 1982-1984. *American Journal of Public Health, 80*(supp.), 61-65.

Haffner, S. M., Diehl, A. K., Mitchell, B. D., Stern, M. P., & Hazuda, H. P. (1990). Increased prevalence of clinical gallbladder disease in subjects with non-insulin-dependent diabetes mellitus. *American Journal of Epidemiology, 132*(2), 327-335.

Harlan, L. C., Bernstein, A. B., & Kessler, L. G. (1991). Cervical cancer screening: Who is not screened and why? *American Journal of Public Health, 81*(7), 885-890.

Hazuda, H. P., Mitchell, B. D., Haffner, S. M., & Stern, M. P. (1991). Obesity in Mexican American subgroups: Findings from the San Antonio Heart Study. *American Journal of Clinical Nutrition, 53*(6 Suppl), 1529S-1534S.

Hollingsworth, D. R., Vaucher, Y., & Yamamoto, T. R. (1991). Diabetes in pregnancy in Mexican Americans. *Diabetes Care, 14*(7), 695-705.

Institute of Medicine. (1994). *Women and health research: Ethical and legal issues of including women in clinical studies.* Washington, DC: National Academy Press.

Kaplan, M. S., & Marks, G. (1990). Adverse effects of acculturation: Psychological distress among Mexican American young adults. *Social Science and Medicine, 31*(12), 1313-1319.

Kirschstein, R. L. (1991). Research on women's health. *American Journal of Public Health, 81*, 291-293.

Leff, M., Orleans, M., Haverkamp, A. D., Baron, A. E., Alderman, B. W., & Freedman, W. L. (1992). The association of maternal low birthweight and infant low birthweight in a racially mixed population. *Paediatrics & Perinatal Epidemiology, 6*(1), 51-61.

Lillie-Blanton, M., Martinez, R. M., Taylor, A. K., & Robinson, B. G. (1993). Latina and African American Women: Continuing disparities in health. *International Journal of Health Services, 23*(3), 555-584.

Marin, B. V., Gomez, C. A., & Tschann, J. M. (1993). Condom use among Hispanic men with secondary female sexual partners. *Public Health Reports, 108*(6), 742-750.

Marin, B. V., Tschann, J. M., Gomez, C. A., & Kegeles, S. M. (1993). Acculturation and gender differences in sexual attitudes and behaviors: Hispanic vs. non-Hispanic White unmarried adults. *American Journal of Public Health, 83*(12), 1259-1261.

Marin, G., Perez-Stable, E. J., & Marin, B. V. (1989). Cigarette smoking among San Francisco Hispanics: The role of acculturation and gender. *American Journal of Public Health, 79*(2), 196-198.

Markides, K. S., & Lee, D. J. (1991). Predictors of health status in middle-aged and older Mexican Americans. *Journal of Gerontology, 46*(5), S243-S249.

Maurer, K. R., Everhart, J. E., Ezzati, T. M., Johannes, R. S., Knowler, W. C., Larson, D. L., Sanders, R., Shawker, T. H., & Roth, H. P. (1989). Prevalence of gallstone disease in the Hispanic populations of the United States. *American Journal of Epidemiology, 131*(5), 836-844.

Menendez, B. S. (1990). AIDS-related mortality among Puerto Rican women in New York City, 1981-1987. *Puerto Rican Health Science Journal, 9*(1), 43-45.

Mitchell, B. D., Haffner, S. M., Hazuda, H. P., Valdez, R., & Stern, M. P. (1992). The relation between serum insulin levels and 8-year changes in lipid, lipoprotein, and blood pressure levels. *American Journal of Epidemiology, 136*(1), 12-22.

Mitchell, B. D., Stern, M. P., Haffner, S. M., Hazuda, H. P., & Patterson, J. K. (1990). Risk factors for cardiovascular mortality in Mexican Americans and non-Hispanic Whites (San Antonio Heart Study). *American Journal of Epidemiology, 131*(3), 423-433.

Moscicki, E. K., Locke, B. Z., Rae, D. S., & Boyd, J. H. (1989). Depressive symptoms among Mexican Americans: The Hispanic Health and Nutrition Examination Survey. *American Journal of Epidemiology, 130*(2), 348-360.

Mosher, W. D., & Aral, S. O. (1991). Testing for sexually transmitted diseases among women of reproductive age: United States, 1988. *Family Planning Perspectives, 23*(5), 216-221.

National Institutes of Health. (1992). *Report of the National Institutes of Health: Opportunities for research on women's health.* Washington, DC: U.S. Department of Health and Human Services.

Novello, A. C., Wise, P. H., & Kleinman D. V. (1991). Hispanic health: Time for data, time for action. *Journal of the American Medical Association, 265,* 253-255.

Nyamathi, A., Bennett, C., Leake, B., Lewis, C., & Flaskerud, J. (1993). AIDS-related knowledge, perceptions, and behaviors among impoverished minority women. *American Journal of Public Health, 83*(1), 65-71.

Oetting, E. R., & Beauvais, F. (1991). Orthogonal cultural identification theory: The cultural identification of adolescents. *International Journal of Addiction, 25*(5A-6A), pp. 655-685).

Ong, K. R., Rubin, S., Brome-Bunting, M., & Labes, K. (1991). Early syphilis in New York City: 1985-1990. *New York State Journal of Medicine, 91*(12), 533-536.

Rassin, D. K., Markides, K. S., Baranowski, T., Bee, D. E., Richardson, C. J., Mikrut, W. D., & Winkler, B. A. (1993). Acculturation and breastfeeding on the United States-Mexico border. *American Journal of Medical Science, 306*(1), 28-34.

Sabogal, F., Faigeles, B., & Catania, J. A. (1993). Data from the National AIDS Behavioral Surveys. II. Multiple sexual partners among Hispanics in high risk cities. *Family Planning Perspectives, 25*(6), 257-262.

Scribner, R., & Dwyer, J. H. (1989). Acculturation and low birthweight among Latinos in the Hispanic HANES. *American Journal of Public Health, 79*(9), 1263-1267.

Siegel, D., Golden, E., Washington, A. E., Morse, S. A., Fullilove, M. T., Catania, J. A., Marin, B., & Hulley, S. B. (1992). Prevalence and correlates of herpes simplex infections. The population-based AIDS in Multiethnic Neighborhoods Study. *Journal of the American Medical Association, 268,* 1702-1708.

Sorenson, S. B., & Telles, C. A. (1991). Self-reports of spousal violence in a Mexican-American and non-Hispanic White population. *Violence and Victimization, 6*(1), 3-15.

Stephen, E., Foote, K., Hendershot, G., & Schoenborn, C. (1994). *Health of the foreign-born population: United States, 1989-1990.* Atlanta, GA: Centers for Disease Control.

U.S. Bureau of the Census. (1991). *The Hispanic population in the United States: March 1991* (Series p-20, No. 455). Washington, DC: U.S. Department of Commerce.

U.S. Department of Health and Human Services. (1991). *Health status of minorities and low-income groups.* Washington, DC: Government Printing Office.

U.S. Office of the Surgeon General. (1993). *One voice, one vision: Recommendations to the Surgeon General to improve Hispanic/Latino health.* Washington, DC: Author.

U.S. Public Health Service. (1985). *Women's health report of the Public Health Service Task Force on Women's Health Issues.* Washington, DC: U.S. Department of Health and Human Services.

Valdez, R. B., Delgado, D. J., Cervantes, R. C., & Bowler, S. (1993). *Cancer in U.S. Latino communities: An exploratory review.* Santa Monica, CA: RAND.

Vega, W. A., Kolody, B., Hwang, J., & Noble, A. (1993). Prevalence and magnitude of perinatal substance exposures in California. *New England Journal of Medicine, 329* (12), 850-854.

Wolfgang, P. E., Semeiks, P. A., & Burnett, W. S. (1991). Cancer incidence in New York City Hispanics, 1982 to 1985. *Ethnicity and Disease, 1*(3), 263-272.

Zambrana, R. E. (1994). The inclusion of Latino women in clinical and research studies: Scientific suggestions for assuring legal and ethical integrity. In Institute of Medicine

(Ed.), *Report on legal and ethical issues relating to the inclusion of women in clinical studies* (pp. 232-240). Washington, DC: National Academy Press.

Zambrana, R. E., Dunkel-Schetter, C., & Scrimshaw, S. (1991). Factors which influence use of prenatal care in low income minority women in Los Angeles. *Journal of Community Health, 16*(5), 283-295.

Zambrana, R. E., Ell, K., Dorrington, C., Wachsman, L., & Hodge, D. (1994). The relationship between psychosocial status and use of emergency pediatric services among immigrant Latino mothers. *Health and Social Work, 19*(2), 93-102.

Zambrana, R. E., Kelly, M., & Raskin, I. (1994). *Patient outcomes and medical effectiveness research: An annotated bibliography related to race, ethnicity, and clinical condition.* Washington, DC: Agency for Health Care policy and Research.

Zhang, J., Markides, K. S., & Lee, D. J. (1991). Health status of diabetic Mexican Americans: Results from the Hispanic HANES. *Ethnicity and Disease, 1*(3), 273-279.

5 Health Issues for Asian/Pacific Island Women

A Brief Overview

GRACE M. WANG

The care of women takes place in the context of the many roles they have in their families, communities, and society. In responding to the diverse and special needs of women in the United States, it is important that health care reform recognize and address the diverse and special needs of the women of the Asian/Pacific Island (A/PI) communities. To best serve these unique constituencies, community-based, bilingual, culturally competent health care services are needed. This discussion will focus on the current knowledge of health care issues involving Asian/Pacific Island women, as well as its limitations.

According to the 1990 U.S. Census, the A/PI population is the fastest growing minority group in the United States. Between 1980 and 1990, the A/PI population increased 108% (Barringer, 1991). Of

AUTHOR'S NOTE: This chapter is based on a presentation made June 13, 1993, at the First National Conference on Cultural Diversity and Women's Health sponsored by the University of Maryland Eastern Shore.

the overall A/PI population, 36% are females over age 20 (Asian & Pacific Islander Data Consortium, 1992). Much of this growth was the result of changes to the immigration laws in the 1960s, as well as refugee resettlement following the war in Indochina. This diverse population includes immigrants from over 20 Asian countries, with many immigrants speaking only their regional dialects. Not surprisingly, the American health care system has not been prepared to meet these very specific linguistic and cultural needs. Moreover, health care professionals have limited information to guide their efforts in providing services to this population.

Health Data/Health Issues

There are few sources of reliable information concerning the A/PI population. Although the National Center for Health Statistics collects vital data from each of the 50 states, much of the information about the health status of Asian/Pacific Islanders is lost in the "other" category. In recent years, states with large A/PI populations have attempted to refine their reporting by attributing data to this general category. But even that is not sufficient because the A/PI population is made up of diverse subgroups. The Asian segment includes, among others, Chinese, Filipino, Japanese, Asian Indian, Korean, Vietnamese, Cambodian, Hmong, Laotian, and Thai peoples. The Pacific Islander segment includes Polynesians, Micronesians, and Melanesians, as well as their respective subgroups.

Data from the National Health Interview survey are often used to guide resource allocation for health promotion and disease prevention. Until recently, however, these surveys were administered in English only (now they are also given in Spanish). Respondents in the A/PI population—those who speak English well enough to participate—typically have been in this country for a longer period of time, and their health beliefs and practices reflect the benefits of mainstream media campaigns. Because not all segments of the Asian/Pacific Island population are represented, an inaccurate picture of the population is recorded. This underrepresentation is exacerbated by the fact that broad-based survey techniques do not consider that

A/PI populations are concentrated in just a very few areas: 70% of the A/PI population resides in only seven states (Leigh, 1994).

Although life expectancy information for A/PI women is not available, data do indicate leading causes of death. Among Chinese Americans, these are heart disease, cancer, cardiovascular disease, and accidents. For Pacific Islanders, the leading causes of death are heart disease, infections, accidents, and alcohol and substance abuse. In addition, obesity is common among native Hawaiians and Samoans (Leigh, 1994).

Much of the other information currently available is based on pooled data, producing results that are misleading and that overlook serious health problems. This information, gathered from the diverse subgroups, results in the erroneous perception of a "healthy minority." For example, according to the National Center for Health Statistics (1991), cancer is the second leading cause of death in the A/PI population, with breast, lung, and cervical cancers being the most common (Leigh, 1994). However, the National Center for Health Statistics also reports that the incidence of breast cancer is much lower in all minority female populations than it is among White females, although data from the California Department of Health clearly indicate that this is not the case. California studies show that Hawaiian women have breast cancer rates in excess of those for White women (Lee, 1992).

National data on the health status of A/PI that promotes the erroneous concept of a healthy minority divert attention from conditions such as tuberculosis and hepatitis, diseases for which immigrant populations are at increased risk due to endemicity in their countries of origin. Dr. Stephen Stellman (1992) of the American Health Foundation compiled mortality data over a 5-year period, using proportional mortality ratios for Chinese and Korean women in New York City. He reports increased proportional mortality ratios among these groups, as compared with White women in New York City, for problems such as tuberculosis and hepatitis B that are common among Asians.

Hepatitis B is of particular importance to women of childbearing age. The Centers for Disease Control 1987 data for perinatal hepatitis B infections indicate a disproportionately high representation of prenatal A/PI women with this disease. Although A/PI women accounted for only 3% of all births nationwide, they represent close to half (48%) of all births to hepatitis B carriers (Leigh, 1994). Because infants exposed through perinatal transmission have the highest rates of infection, screening and newborn follow-up for immunizations are the cornerstone of disease prevention in the A/PI population. Re- sources for these efforts are a priority.

The Asian/Pacific Islander information sheet from the National Heart, Lung, and Blood Institute reports that the poverty rate for this group is lower than that for the total U.S. population (National Institutes of Health, 1992). However, data from the 1990 Census show that 11.9% of A/PI families live below the poverty level, compared to 10.3% of the total population (Lin-Fu, 1994). In addition, income for the A/PI population follows a bimodal distribution. A sizable percentage of newly arrived Asian/Pacific Islanders work in the service industry, often in poorly paid jobs such as food service, cleaning, and household work; those who have been in the United States for longer periods have higher levels of income and education (Lin-Fu, 1988).

Local data from areas with large A/PI populations provide insight into factors that have an impact on socioeconomic status, as well as a more accurate assessment of health status. The 1990 U.S. Census data on Asian/Pacific Islanders in New York City show that this population has the greatest proportion of linguistically isolated households, those in which no one over the age of 14 speaks English "well" or "very well" (Asian & Pacific Islander Data Consortium, 1992). This one factor certainly has implications in a variety of areas, including earning potential.

Access to Care

Data that erroneously depict a healthy model minority result in resource allocations that ultimately diminish access to health care services. *Healthy People 2000,* which contains the blueprint for the nation's health in the year 2000, is a federal document containing 637 objectives (U.S. Department of Health & Human Services, 1990). Only 10 of these objectives address the health needs of the A/PI population. (Of those, the objective to reduce smoking among Southeast Asian men is repeated three times.)

Several surveys of Asian women have demonstrated the need for more effective means to promote access to care, indicating that mainstream health education efforts have had little impact on non-English speaking communities. Indeed, the biomedical approach, with its emphasis on disease, does not address the problem of access to care—a major health consideration for many women in the A/PI community.

Asian Health Services, a community health center in Oakland, California, has reported on the impact of linguistic, cultural, and financial barriers to health care in the Chinese community. The data for this study were collected from home interviews, using a bilingual survey with modified questions from the CDC Behavioral Risk Factor Survey. The investigators found that Chinese females 40 and older who were not fluent in English were significantly less likely to have heard of mammograms than those who spoke English. Similarly, those who were not English speakers were more likely to delay screening for cervical and breast cancer than those who were fluent in English. About 50% of the women over age who were fluent in English had had their last mammogram within the past 2 years; only 21% of those not fluent in English had had a mammogram during the same time period. The investigators cross-tabbed health behavior with income and found that women with higher incomes were more likely to have knowledge of mammograms than those with household incomes below $10,000 per year. In addition, 44% of those in the higher bracket knew what a Pap smear was, whereas only 22% of women below poverty level were familiar with this procedure (Chen et al., 1992).

The Korean Health Survey in Los Angeles found that only 29% of women over age 18 had had a breast exam within the previous year, compared to 50% of all American women (Han, 1990). Only 35% of the women surveyed had ever had a Pap smear, as compared with one half of all U.S. women. Christopher Jenkins, in his studies at the University of California at San Francisco on cancer risk and preventive practices among Vietnamese refugees, found that only 17% of Vietnamese women over age 40 had ever had a mammogram (Jenkins, McPhee, Bird, & Bonilla, 1990). He also compared cancer-screening practices in the Vietnamese community with those of the general population and found that high rates of nonuse had serious implications for health outcomes. These findings demonstrate the need for community-based, bilingual, culturally competent health care services for the women of immigrant communities.

Recommendations

The Chinatown Health Clinic, a federally funded community health center in New York City, presents a model for community-based health service delivery for women in A/PI communities. The clinic provides bilingual primary health care services to indigent recent immigrants in the New York City Chinese community. Current programs integrate health education and outreach in order to promote preventive health practices. The clinic offers mammography vouchers to offset the cost of this procedure and translation assistance to make offsite mammography services accessible to clinic patients. Health education efforts include community outreach at health fairs, workplace screening activities, and newspaper articles and radio presentations in the Chinese language media.

Epilogue

In the current atmosphere of health care reform, it is important to advocate data collection that recognizes the diversity within the A/PI population. This, in turn, will better identify the specific needs that must be addressed, such as the necessity of community-based programs that are responsive to the women of this unique population. Bilingual, culturally competent services with specific programs for health education and outreach must be the standard of care in A/PI communities.

References

Asian & Pacific Islander Data Consortium. (1992). *Asian and Pacific Islander American Profile Series 1A*. New York: Author. (Available from Asian & Pacific Islander

American Health Forum, 116 New Montgomery Street, Suite 531, San Francisco, California 94105. 415/541-0866).

Barringer, F. (1991, March 11). Census shows profound change in racial makeup of the nation. *New York Times*, p. 1.

Chen, A., Lew, R., Thai, V., Ko, K. L., Okahara, L., Hirota, S., Chan, S., Wong, W., Saika, G., Folkers, L. F., & Marquez, B. (1992, April 24). Behavioral risk factor survey of Chinese-California. *Morbidity and Mortality Weekly Reports, 41*, 266-270.

Han, E. (1990, November 17). *Korean health survey in Southern California: A preliminary report on health status and health care needs of Korean immigrants*. Paper presented at the Asian American Health Forum conference, A/PI: Dispelling the Myth of a Healthly Minority, in Bethesda, MD.

Jenkins, C., McPhee, S., Bird, J., & Bonilla, N. (1990). Cancer risks and prevention behaviors among Vietnamese refugees. *Western Journal of Medicine, 153*, 34-39.

Lee, M. (1992). *Breast and cervical cancer in Asian and Pacific Islander women*. San Francisco: Asian & Pacific Islander American Health Forum.

Leigh, W. A. (1994). The health status of women of color. In C. Costello & A. J. Stone (Eds.), *The American woman 1994-95: Where we stand* (pp. 154-196). New York: Norton.

Lin-Fu, J. S. (1988). Population characteristics and health care needs of Asian Pacific Americans. *Public Health Reports, 103*, 18-27.

Lin-Fu, J. S. (1994). Asian and Pacific Islander Americans: An overview of demographic characteristics and health issues. *Asian American and Pacific Islander Journal of Health, 2*, 20-36.

National Center for Health Statistics. (1991). *Health, United States, 1990*. Hyattsville, MD: Public Health Service.

National Institutes of Health. (1992). Data on Asian/Pacific Islanders. (Available from NHLBI Education Programs Information Center, P.O. Box 30105, Bethesda, MD 20824-0105. 301/951-3160)

Stellman, S. (1992, September 17). Poster presented at the American College of Epidemiology, Bethesda, MD.

U.S. Department of Health & Human Services, Public Health Service. (1990). *Healthy people 2000. National health promotion and disease prevention objectives* (DHHS Publication No. (PHS) 91-50213). Washington, DC: Government Printing Office.

6 Domestic Violence in Asian/Pacific Island Communities
A Public Health Issue

PATRICIA ENG

Domestic violence is a national health epidemic that occurs in every community and claims half of this nation's women as direct victims. Battered women of color and immigrant women face specific barriers placing them at further risk. This chapter will focus specifically on Asian immigrant women who are confronted with economic, cultural, and institutional barriers to affordable and culturally sensitive health care.

Information is drawn from the work of the New York Asian Women's Center, a grassroots, community-based program focusing on battering and other forms of violence against women in the Asian community. It offers the first 24-hour Asian multilingual hot line and shelter program on the East Coast for Asian battered women. The center assists women who have sustained injuries both physically and mentally over many years. Counselors at the center often link women and accompany them to health care professionals, working closely with community health facilities to ensure that women do not fall through the cracks.

Although domestic violence is not new to Asian communities across the United States, organized community responses to this problem are fairly new. Only a few shelter programs are designed to work with Asian immigrant battered women. Most of these programs are situated in large urban areas where substantial Asian populations exist, such as Los Angeles, San Francisco, Boston, Chicago, and New York. Although each program is unique in its particular setting, the problems that battered women face when reaching out to each of the programs are similar.

Case Histories

Woman abuse is a national health epidemic and has a devastating impact on women in the Asian/Pacific Island (A/PI) communities. Two case histories are offered to illustrate this point.

THE STORY OF WAI

Wai is a Chinese immigrant woman who has been abused by her husband for the past 18 years. Throughout her marriage, she has been defecated on, slapped, punched, raped, threatened with death, and routinely belittled and humiliated. Wai has three children, who have witnessed many of these abusive incidents. As an immigrant woman, she rarely turned to the health care system (except when her children needed health care), nor did anyone stop to ask her about the violence she was experiencing.

With nowhere to turn, Wai internalized the abuse. Believing that somehow she caused the abuse, Wai's self-esteem dwindled, her ability to concentrate on most tasks was lost, and she was finally certified as disabled from an employment standpoint. By this time, she had been evaluated by the health care system as needing medications, relying on these drugs to function. The abuse grew so intolerable that she became suicidal.

Wai contacted the New York Asian Women's Center, a program for battered women in the Asian community, that, in turn, intervened by referring her for psychiatric evaluation. She became angry at the center because of a tremendous stigma attached to mental health problems. Wai felt totally humiliated in the eyes of her community.

After her hospitalization, Wai was seen on an outpatient basis at a local mental health program in order to continue her prescribed medication. Although she complained that the medication was giving her headaches, Wai was extremely reluctant to speak with the psychiatrist about adjusting her prescription.

A counselor from the New York Asian Women's Center had accompanied Wai to her psychiatrist's office and heard him berate her, blaming her for the "mess" her family was in. He told her that she was wasting his time and that of the other professionals. This psychiatrist was Chinese, and he felt culturally justified in saying these things to her. Unfortunately, it is not uncommon for women to be asked questions that imply they somehow provoked the violence.

THE STORY OF KAM

Kam is a 29-year-old woman who was physically and verbally abused by her husband throughout their 3-year marriage. After a particularly brutal incident, she was treated for her injuries by a private physician in the community. A few weeks later, she returned to the doctor for documentation in order to help her obtain an Order of Protection. The doctor demanded a fee of $100 to provide her with a copy of her medical record.

Having paid the $100, Kam obtained the Order of Protection and got her own apartment. Soon after, she was brutally assaulted by her husband, who had been stalking her. He assaulted her with a hammer, much in the style of a widely publicized case that had occurred a year earlier, also involving a Chinese immigrant man who beat his wife with a hammer. The woman in that case died and the man in that case was sentenced to 5 years probation with no jail time. Kam was so upset by this attack that she began expressing suicidal thoughts.

Background

As the Asian population in the United States grows, so too do the number of incidences of violence against Asian women. Each year, countless Asian women are "sold" into the country as mail-order brides, countless rapes go unreported, and incest, the greatest taboo of all, remains hidden in the community's darkest closets. In the early 1980s, the New York City Department of Health Statistics indicated that the suicide rate among Chinese women was three times greater than that among Chinese men.

Battering occurs with alarming regularity within the Asian community, just as it does in the larger American society. Each year, the New York Asian Women's Center alone receives over 3,000 calls from battered women across the country who are bitten, punched, stabbed, and shot. They are threatened with knives or guns and denied food and money. They are verbally harassed and sexually assaulted. They are also killed.

Each year, newspaper accounts tell us about women and children in the Asian community who die at the hands of their abusers or who take their own lives in order to escape the violence. Unfortunately, the case histories presented here are not unique, nor are they the most horrendous. Women often turn to others for help, perhaps only subtly hinting at violence, but those cries for help are unheard or ignored. If these cries left unheard, other physical symptoms may appear, such as sleeping and eating disorders, inability to concentrate, headaches, and other unexplained physical symptoms. Many of the women who contact the New York Asian Women's Center complain about health problems of this nature, which have persisted since the abuse began.

NATIONAL OVERVIEW

Woman abuse is a national health epidemic that has never been defined as such. In 1985, the U.S. Surgeon General reported that battering was the single greatest cause of injury to women, more common than auto accidents, muggings, and rape combined.

The statistics are staggering:

- It is estimated that half of the women in the United States are abused by their partners (Schulman, 1979; Straus, Gelles, & Steinmetz, 1980). The FBI estimates that one woman is being battered every 15 seconds.
- The FBI reported in 1990 that about 30% of the women who are killed each year are the victims of husbands or boyfriends.

- It has been estimated that as many as 35% of all women treated in emergency rooms have injuries from abusive partners (American Medical Association, 1992).

Woman abuse claims half of this nation's women as direct victims and the other half indirectly as the concerned daughters, mothers, sisters, or friends of the victims. It affects every community in this country (Straus et al., 1980). It is exacerbated by other economic, cultural, and institutional barriers in areas such as employment, housing, child care, and immigration, as well as other legal issues that prevent access to affordable and culturally sensitive health care. It touches upon every aspect of a woman's life: what she says, how she dresses, where she works, who she associates with, and even what sex her children are. It doesn't matter whether she has any control over these matters or not; she is made to feel that she is somehow responsible. One study estimated that domestic violence accounts for as much as $10 billion in health and social welfare costs (Meyer, 1992).

According to the national crime survey completed by the U.S. Department of Justice in 1982, once a woman has been victimized by domestic violence, she is likely to be revictimized. During a 6-month period following an incident of domestic violence, approximately 32% of the women were battered again. In addition, 48% of all incidents of domestic violence against women discovered in the survey were not reported to the police.

Battered women visit primary care physicians for a variety of medical complaints, such as headaches, sleep disorders, depression, and abdominal pain (Stark et al., 1981). According to one study, 64% of hospitalized female psychiatric patients had a history of being physically abused as an adult (Jacobsen & Richardson, 1987). Studies conducted by Stark and Flitcraft also indicated a strong correlation between women who attempted suicide and domestic violence (American Medical Association, 1992) and an even stronger correlation (50%) among Black women (Flitcraft & Stark, 1986). Child abuse and domestic violence are also related; as many as 59% of mothers of abused children were themselves battered (American Medical Association, 1992). In fact, battering often begins or escalates during pregnancy. One source indicates that as many as 37% of all pregnant women are abused (Helton & Snodgrass, 1987). The American Medical Association estimates that women who are battered are twice as likely to miscarry and four times more likely to deliver a low birth weight baby (March of Dimes, 1993).

Although many battered women require medical attention, few women who use the health care system are ever identified as victims of, or receive help with, domestic violence. Lacking sufficient training, health care providers historically have not recognized battered women who seek help. Doctors are not trained to take responsibility for treating domestic violence beyond the physical injuries. Therefore, despite inconsistencies in stated causes or explanations, health care providers do not probe into the true nature of the injuries (Smolowe, 1992). As a result, many battered women are often characterized as "hysterical" or treated with tranquilizers and other drugs.

As domestic violence awareness increases, hospitals nationwide have begun to place domestic violence protocols on file, but more often than not, such protocols are never fully implemented. Patients are not routinely asked about how injuries were sustained, nor are they asked in a confidential setting away from the batterer. Intake forms do not include questions on domestic violence, nor are injuries photographed, even when identified as domestic abuse. Health care providers are clearly reluctant to identify or become involved in issues of family violence.

DOMESTIC VIOLENCE IN ASIAN COMMUNITIES

Health issues in A/PI communities have historically been identified generically, without regard to gender differences. Of course, in this scenario, the net effect is that women's specific health issues are marginalized and invisible. When women's health issues in the Asian Pacific community are isolated, we find distressing statistics:

- Breast cancer is by far the most commonly occurring cancer among A/PI women, yet 70% of Asian women surveyed never had a mammogram (Lee, 1992).
- Even though Asian women are most likely of all women of color to have health insurance, they are the least likely to have an annual physical exam. Asian women are least likely to ever have a Pap smear or a mammogram (Communications Consortium, 1991).

- Elderly Chinese and Japanese women have the highest suicide rate of all ethnic groups, including Whites (Lin-Fu, 1988).

When this information is combined with the statistics on battering, we get disastrous results.

Battering exists in the Asian Pacific/Islander community just as it does in every segment of our society. The difference is in the options (or rather, lack of them) available to immigrant women. We cannot focus on health needs of Asian battered women without also looking at the numerous other factors that prevent them from accessing health care.

For example, tradition is such that Asian women are held responsible for the success of their marriages. For Asian women, failure in marriage is not only an individual failure but also a source of shame and humiliation for the entire family. Women who reveal family problems to outsiders are looked upon harshly by the community. For these reasons, getting help from anyone outside the family or leaving the relationship are not acceptable options for many Asian women. To confront the violence is often synonymous with condemning herself to isolation and ostracism.

Many Asian women are faced with problems of being immigrant women; they often depend socially and economically on the Asian community in which they live or work. Many do not possess the English-language skills needed in order to survive outside of the Asian community, and, as a result, their social networks are limited. These women are not able to negotiate systems or institutions beyond the borders of the community, and, as a result, they are trapped in violent situations. Often their abusers speak better English and therefore are better able to convince others that the women are "crazy" or the source of the problems. Their children are often in bilingual education programs that do not exist outside of the community, thus compelling women to remain where they are, in violent relationships.

U.S. immigration laws are such that many immigrant women arrive without members of their own families, leaving them prey to the violence from abusive husbands and their husbands' relatives. Immigrant women often suffer at the hands of multiple abusers when family members on the abuser's side join in the violence or, at best, collude with the batterer in inflicting violence or withholding food, money, and other essentials. This information also shatters myths and stereotypes about the Asian community's harmonious family image, often held up as a prototype or model of family support.

Immigration laws also have been used to leave women in dangerous, often life-threatening relationships. Some women arrive in this country through marriage to a U.S. citizen or permanent resident on a "conditional resident" status. After 2 years, the couple must file a joint petition with the Immigration and Naturalization Service (INS) to obtain lawful status for the wife. Batterers invariably use this power, granted to them by INS, to deliberately render their victims undocumented and completely powerless.

This is only one example of how institutions effectively collude with abusers to gain complete control over their victims, leaving these women with little or no means to defend themselves or to challenge the violent behavior. Therefore, a woman who chooses to leave her husband may be facing the choice of abandoning her entire community or risking the danger of retaliation from the abuser and/or his family. Battered Asian immigrant women are fearful of jeopardizing their own legal status or any chance of petitioning relatives to come to the United States if they take any action to confront their abuser's violent behavior. Asian women have few support systems to start with, but what they have may be taken away if they choose to challenge the violence in their lives.

The disadvantaged economic position of women is exacerbated by Asian women's immigrant status. In restaurants, garment factories, and commercial businesses, women are relegated to the lowest-paying jobs, many paying below the minimum wage. These jobs are often seasonal and afford little job security. However, due to language differences and lack of marketable skills, most women can find employment only within the borders of the Asian community. Some women do "homework," the piecing together of fabric or jewelry that is brought to their homes. Moving away from the community means an instant loss of livelihood for them. Even a temporary leave of absence from these jobs in order to maintain their personal safety or the safety of their children may cost women their jobs.

Under such circumstances, more than half of the women who contact the Asian Women's Center each year never receive medical attention for their injuries. Many Asian women use health care facilities only in dire emergencies. This is consistent with the Asian community's limited use of health care facilities in general. Economically, few immigrant families have comprehensive health insurance. Culturally, some community residents prefer Eastern health remedies, which may be more consistent with their diets. Western health care facilities are used by Asian immigrants only when symptoms have become quite serious. Hospitals, in the eyes of many community members, are associated with death and to be avoided at all costs.

The only time Asian immigrant women have ongoing health care is when they are pregnant. However, as previously noted, battering often starts or escalates in severity during pregnancy. Such gruesome statistics are confirmed through numerous referrals received by the New York Asian Women's Center from a local prenatal clinic serving primarily Asian immigrant women. In these situations, it is often hard to engage the women, because they are often accompanied by the expectant fathers. Many women are not ready to deal with the violence when doing so could result in becoming a single parent. These women may hope that the baby's birth will begin a new life for the family and erase the violence from their lives.

When women do turn to health care providers specifically for injuries, they generally feel more comfortable seeing physicians in the Asian community. However, many private physicians do not want to take part in documenting abuses, because of personal biases, fear of legal involvement, and inconvenience. For example, one woman who was repeatedly beaten by her husband was concerned about her child, who also was abused. She took the child to a private physician in the community and asked him to file a report with child welfare authorities. The doctor told her that she would need to see a different physician to file such a report.

Many women tend to stay away from medical institutions because of a well-founded fear that their children may be taken away from them if they reveal any problems of family violence. Kim, a Korean woman who was pregnant from her abusive boyfriend, carried her pregnancy to term because she feared his violence. When the child was born, child welfare workers, called in by the hospital, immediately placed the child in foster care until Kim agreed to live apart from her boyfriend and not to see him.

Recommendations

In summary, domestic violence is a dangerous health care problem for Asian women. Health remedies must take into consideration societal factors such as immigration laws, economics, and cultural considerations, all of which infringe upon the choices that women have available to them.

Health care providers must receive training in the area of domestic violence to understand the issues and to identify and assist battered women who seek medical care. They must be trained to ask questions and more fully document cases of domestic violence. It is no longer possible for doctors to treat simply the symptoms of domestic violence. Medical practitioners must expand their treatment to offer true relief and prevention of further injury to the bodies and souls of all battered women.

Clearly, there is a need for more bilingual, bicultural health care workers who understand their responsibility extends beyond treatment of injuries and symptoms to offering choices, taking the time to go over safety plans with women, and connecting them with other agencies in the community. It is imperative that women are given control over their own lives and allowed to make choices for themselves, rather than having that control taken away, as is common in a medical setting.

It is time that we no longer marginalize the health, and very lives, of Asian Pacific women. It is time that we bring good health and safety home to all women.

References

American Medical Association. (1992, June). *Diagnostic and treatment guidelines on domestic violence*. Chicago: Author.

Communications Consortium & National Council of Negro Women. (1991). *Women of color reproductive health poll*. Washington, DC: Author.

Flitcraft, A., & Stark, E. (1986). Woman battering, a prevention oriented approach. In *The physician assistant's guide to health promotion and disease prevention* (pp. 56-74). Atlanta, GA: Emory School of Medicine.

Helton, A., & Snodgrass, F. (1987, September). Battering during pregnancy. *Birth, 14*, 3.

Jacobsen, A., & Richardson, B. (1987). Assault experiences of 100 psychiatric patients: Evidence of the need for routine inquiry. *American Journal of Psychiatry, 144,* 908-913.

Lee, M. (1992). Breast and cervical cancer in Asian and Pacific Islander women. *Asian American Health Forum Focus, 3,* 2.

Lin-Fu, J. S. (1988, January). Population characteristics and health needs of Asian Pacific Americans. *Public Health Reports, 103,* 18-27.

March of Dimes. (1993, June 23). *Request for proposal from Andronike Tasamas for campaign for healthier babies.* Document on file, National Center on Women and Family Law, New York.

Meyer, H. (1992, January 6). The billion dollar epidemic. *American Medical News,* p. 7.

Schulman, M. A. (1979). *A survey on spousal violence against women in Kentucky* (Study No. 70927001). Lexington: Kentucky Commission on Women.

Smolowe, J. (1992, June 29). What the doctor should do. *Time Magazine,* p. 57.

Stark, E., Flitcraft, A., Zuckerman, D., Grey, A., Robison, J., & Franzier, W. (1981). *Wife abuse in the medical setting: An introduction for health personnel.* Washington, DC: Office of Domestic Violence.

Straus, M. A., Gelles, R. D., & Steinmetz, S. K. (1980). *Behind closed doors: Violence in American families.* New York: Anchor/Doubleday.

7 Mental Health Issues of Asian/Pacific Island Women

REIKO HOMMA TRUE

Although women's health and mental health issues are now beginning to attract national concerns in the United States, little support has been given so far to identify minority women's mental health needs, including those of Asian/Pacific Island (A/PI) women, or to provide funding for services that are culturally appropriate for their needs.

American society treats mental health issues with a general lack of understanding and reluctance. In the case of A/PI women, this is exacerbated by other factors:

The relatively small number of people, and the perception that their needs are of lesser significance or nonexistent

The wide geographic distribution and diverse nature of the A/PI population, which creates methodological problems for epidemiological needs assessment and other research investigations

Perceptions of Asian Americans as a model minority with few problems, particularly related to mental illness or psychological distress

Until recently, A/PI leaders themselves were reluctant to focus on the possible existence of mental health issues in their communities. Their reluctance was partly due to the cultural stigma of mental illness, but they were also strongly influenced by their fear of attracting more negative publicity about their communities when they have already suffered persistent racism and hostility from the dominant groups for many years. However, as a result of a growing awareness about women's issues, an emerging group of A/PI women, from both professional and community groups, is beginning to speak out and identify the unique mental health needs and problems faced by their compatriots. The goal of this chapter is to review the information available to date and to help readers develop greater cultural understanding about the needs of A/PI women.

Demographic Profile

Although they are viewed by the U.S. public as a fairly homogenous group, the umbrella term *Asian and Pacific Islander women* covers a diverse group, representing as many as 27 Asian American and over 30 Pacific Islander groups, including Chinese, Filipinos, Japanese, Koreans, East Indians, and Southeast Asians, as well as Hawaiians, Samoans, and Guamanians. The 1990 U. S. census counted over 7.27 million Asians and Pacific Islanders, of whom 3.715 million (51% of the population) were women.

A/PI women are on average older than men, with a median age of 31.8 years, compared to 29.0 years for males, reflecting the generally longer life expectancy of females in the United States. Although data are not available by sex, it is important to note that 65.6% of all Asians are foreign born and 75.4% speak a language other than English at home. Although Pacific Islanders have a lower percentage of foreign born (12%), subgroup variations include 60.9% foreign-born Tongans and 77.9% foreign-born Melanesians (U.S. Bureau of the Census, 1992).

Although most A/PI women are married, Census Bureau (1992) data indicate that as of March 1991, 26% had never married, 8% were widowed, and 6% were divorced, compared to 28%, 2.5%, and 7% of white women, respectively. Whereas the percentage of all U.S. households headed by females was 16.5% in 1990, the figure for Asians was

12%. However, 26.2% of Cambodian households had female heads (U.S. Bureau of the Census, 1993). Overall educational achievement by A/PI women was high (74% high school graduates or higher, 31.8% with bachelor's degree or more), compared to the general U.S. population (74.8% and 17.6%), but there was great subgroup variability. Those from rural areas had the least education—the percentages of Hmong, Cambodians, and Laotians with a high school diploma or more were 19%, 25.3%, and 29.8% respectively (U.S. Bureau of the Census, 1993).

Most adult Asian (60%) and Pacific Islander (62.5%) women were in the labor force, compared to 56.8% of all total U.S. women, but the rates for some refugee groups were very low (19.9% for Hmong, 37.3% for Cambodians, and 49.5% for Laotians). The median earnings of A/PI women in 1990 was $21,320, higher than for white women ($20,050). However, the figure masks a great variability, with some women working as highly trained managers and professionals, and others earning marginal wages as sweatshop seamstresses or hotel maids. Of those below poverty level, 36% were in female-headed households (U.S. Bureau of the Census, 1993).

Historical Background

Because of laws restricting entry by women in the early years of Asian immigration, the number of women was small to start. However, as the immigration laws were revised to permit families to immigrate together and wives to rejoin their husbands, the number of Asian women immigrants increased rapidly, and they now outnumber men by 158,000.

Historically, the first group of Asian women to immigrate were the Chinese, who arrived nearly 150 years ago in the mid-1800s. Because of the prohibitive cost of the long journey from China and the traditional reluctance to send women overseas, only a small number of women were able to accompany their husbands at the early stage of Chinese immigration. Before more Chinese women had the chance to enter the United States, strong anti-Chinese sentiment erupted after Chinese male laborers began to achieve some level of economic success in various enterprises. The Chinese were quickly perceived as potential threats to the socioeconomic security of the white Americans, and exclusionary immigration laws were created, beginning in 1882, to severely limit further entry of Chinese, including women. In their place, a large number of Japanese males were brought in as cheap laborers to fill the back-breaking jobs no one else wanted. The Japanese government actively encouraged the immigration of women as wives of male laborers, a strategy for preventing problems endemic to bachelor societies, such as prostitution, violence, and gambling. Although the Japanese immigrants were subsequently perceived as a new threat, a significant number of Japanese women settled in the United States with their husbands before the restrictions were extended to them through the National Origins Act in 1924 (Nakano, 1990).

The groups that followed the Chinese and Japanese were Korean and Filipino laborers. However, in the early 1900s, their number was relatively small, and the number of women who came with their husbands was small until recently (Takaki, 1989).

In 1965, the immigration laws were significantly liberalized to permit increased numbers of immigrants from Asian countries and to allow the reunion of family members, including wives who had been separated from their husbands for many years. This made it possible for a large number of Chinese, Filipino, and Korean women to bring their families and rejoin husbands (Lee, 1985; Navarro, 1976; Yung 1986).

After the end of the Vietnam War in 1975, a large wave of Southeast Asian refugee women were forced to flee their countries, and many of them resettled in the United States with their families (Tien, 1994). More recently, immigration from the Indian subcontinent is also increasing (Jayakar, 1994).

Because of these historical differences, there are important diversities among the A/PI women. For example, although there are significant numbers of fourth- or fifth-generation, U.S.-born Japanese- and Chinese-American women, at least 63% of Asian Americans are foreign born. The differences among subgroups are dramatic: Nearly 80% of Vietnamese, Laotians, and Cambodians are foreign born, compared to only 32% of Japanese Americans (U.S. Bureau of the Census, 1993).

Extent and Nature of
Mental Health Problems

Prevalence Data. In the absence of comprehensive epidemiological data on the mental health status of Asians and Pacific Islanders in the United States, regardless of gender, information specific to A/PI women is virtually nonexistent. Most policymakers did not support the effort to make this information a priority for investigation, tending to assume that A/PI people had few mental health problems, and that families and community would prefer to take care of those who did.

It may be helpful to review some findings from epidemiological studies conducted in Asia, mainly in Japan, China, and Taiwan. Some studies were modeled after the epidemiological studies attempted in the United States in the 1950s and 1960s, designed to be quite extensive for certain defined geographic regions. The findings from these studies were cross-tabulated by gender and provide information concerning the extent or prevalence of mental health problems among women in the area. To some extent, these data may be applicable to A/PI women in the United States. For example, Lin, Rin, Yeh, Hsu, and Chu (1969) investigated the prevalence of various categories of mental illness in three communities in Taiwan in 1963 and found an overall rate for all mental disorders for men and women to be 16.1 and 18.3 per 1,000, respectively. Although the difference in overall rates for the sexes was not statistically significant, there were significant differences within subcategories: high rates of mental deficiency and psychopathic personality for males; high rates of psychoneuroses for women, particularly in middle to older age. Also of note was a significantly higher incidence of schizophrenia among the 51 to 60 (7.1) and 61 to 70-year-old women (7.8) than among men in the same age groups (2.5 and 2.0 respectively). The overall findings seem to correspond to those of the epidemiological studies in the United States, in which women had higher rates of affective disorders, panic/ obsessive-compulsive disorders, somatization, and phobias, apparently subsumed under the diagnosis of psychoneuroses in Lin et al.'s investigation. The higher rate of antisocial personality disorder for men in U.S. studies also corresponds with the Taiwan study's psychopathic personality (Robbins, Locke, & Regier, 1991).

In the absence of national data on A/PI women, it is helpful to consider the implications of some of the regional data about their mental health. For example, Ying (1988) attempted to explore the level of depressive symptomatology among San Francisco-based Chinese Americans through a telephone survey using the Center for Epidemiological Studies-Depression Scale (CES-D). Among the 360 subjects who agreed to be interviewed, 182 were women. Their mean depression score was 12.83, somewhat higher than the mean score of 10.25 for men. The score was also considerably higher than the mean score (ranging from 7.94 to 9.25) for a predominantly white sample in a study by Radloff (1977). Among the general population, a CES-D mean of 16 and above was used to indicate clinical depression. In the sample reported by Radloff for the white population, 19% scored 16 or above, whereas 24% of the Ying's (1988) combined male and female sample scored 16 or above. Ying also found that those who belonged to a lower socioeconomic level (as measured by education and occupation) scored as significantly more depressed than those who were at higher socioeconomic levels.

In a study in Chicago, Hurh and Kim (1990) conducted diagnostic interviews with 622 Korean immigrants (20 years and older) to explore the extent of mental health problems among more recent immigrants, using the CES-D scale, the Health Opinion Survey (HOS), and the Memorial University of Newfoundland Scale of Happiness (MUNSH). Their findings indicated that those who were married, highly educated, and currently employed in a high-status occupation indicated better subjective mental health than others. They also found significant gender differences in that the correlates for mental health for males were a set of work-related variables, whereas family life satisfaction and several ethnic attachment variables were moderately related for females.

Among Asian immigrant groups, it is generally agreed that Southeast Asian refugees face the greatest stress in adjusting to a new life in the United States. Many women suffered traumatic experiences and major losses of close family members before their immigration and frequently experience recurring symptoms of posttraumatic stress disorder (PTSD) (Rumbaut, 1985). In a statewide needs assessment study in California, Gong-Guy (1987) found that refugees from rural areas such as Cambodia and Laos, who had little previous exposure to modern urban living, were particularly ill-prepared for large, complex urban communities and were often experiencing significant psychiatric symptoms, such as high levels of depression, anxiety, and various psychosocial dysfunctions (difficulty performing tasks of daily living, school, or work). Among the refugee groups, Cambodians were exposed to the most atrocities and had to remain in camps much longer than others. Using the data from Gong-Guy's study (1987), Chung (1991) examined the gender and subgroup differences among the refugees—Cambodians, Laotians, and Vietnamese —and found that women in all three groups were more distressed than men. Among the three groups, she found that the Cambodians were the most distressed, followed by Laotians and Vietnamese.

The experience of Cambodian women refugees in Long Beach, California, reported by Rozee and Van Boemel (1989), provided a glimpse into the harrowing experience of war trauma and abuse suffered by older Cambodian women. The researchers conducted a series of supportive group services for refugee women who were diagnosed as functionally blind without organic basis, and therefore could not qualify for disability assistance. Among them, 90% reported losing 1 to 10 relatives and witnessing the massacre of family members. It was almost as if their traumas were so great that they did not wish to see anything; they suffered from severe depression, nightmares, sleep disturbances, and other symptoms associated with PTSD.

Another group of Asian Pacific Americans who were subjected to significant trauma were Japanese Americans, who were labeled enemy aliens in the United States during World War II and confined in concentration camps, euphemistically called "internment camps." The experience of being uprooted from their own homes, labeled enemy aliens even when they were born in the United States, deprived of their civil rights, and subjected to subhuman conditions was devastating to most Japanese Americans. Although most tried to rebuild their lives after the war, many carried lasting psychic scars, such as a pervasive sense of insecurity, depression, and low self-esteem. In her interview of third-generation Japanese Americans, many of whom were women, Nagata (1991) identified how the psychological trauma, humiliation, and fears about future persecution were passed on to subsequent generations of Japanese Americans, even though they were not personally subjected to the trauma.

Utilization Data. Although mental health service utilization data are often accepted as a measure of the level of mental health problems present in communities, they provide little help in understanding the problems in the A/PI community; their record of service use has traditionally been very low (Snowden & Cheung, 1990; Sue & McKinney, 1975). For example, while the A/PI population constitutes 9.5% of the total in California (1990 Census), their statewide use of community mental health services during fiscal year 1989-1990 was 4.29% (2.32% for women; 1.97% for men) (California Department of Mental Health, 1992).

The San Francisco Community Mental Health Services showed 10.8% A/PI clients during the same period. Although this use figure represents a significant improvement over the past 15 years, made possible through the concerted effort of service providers to develop culturally sensitive, bilingual programs, it still represents underuse of mental health services by Asian Pacific citizens, who constitute 25% of the city's total population.

Some factors affecting low service use are thought to include

fear of establishment authorities;

absence of bilingual, culturally sensitive service providers;

cultural stigma among Asians about mental illness, creating family shame to acknowledge having psychiatric problems;

traditional reluctance to seek outside help;

cost of seeking help; and

institutional barriers such as geographic location or hours of operation.

Recognizing that the mental health problems in A/PI communities were much more extensive, community leaders and mental health professionals in key communities began to advocate for and develop programs that were more culturally responsive (President's Commission on Mental Health, 1978). For this reason, in some communities that made the effort to be more responsive, service use by A/PI clients has increased significantly (Sue, 1988). Although research about the gender differences among Asian American mental health clients is still limited, the usage data from Los Angeles and San Francisco counties in California provide some information.

As part of the extensive Los Angeles County Mental Health Service data analysis at the National Research Center on Asian American Mental Health, Fujino and Chung (1991) analyzed the gender differences in rates of psychiatric disorders among four ethnic groups of mental health clients. Besides confirming previous studies showing that Asian Americans tended to under use available services, the authors also found significant gender differences in rates of psychiatric disorders among the Asian American users of mental health services: Males (19.8%) significantly outnumbered females (10.4%) in the schizophrenic diagnosis, whereas females (21.2%) were more likely to suffer depressive disorder than males (15.1%). The rate for anxiety disorder among Asian males was higher than among females, 8.3% versus 7.4%. Although adjustment disorder was greater among female patients, the difference was not statistically significant.

Medical Service Utilization. In their review of U.S. women's mental health service use data, Mowbray and Benedek (1988) noted that a significantly greater number of women went to primary care physicians for help with their emotional problems. When Yu, Liu, & Wong (1987) reviewed the use data of a Chinatown health clinic in Boston, they also found that a significant number of Chinese women seen at the clinic were being treated for symptoms related to depression.

Additional support for this trend was also identified by Ying (1990), when she conducted a survey in San Francisco on the help-seeking attitude of Chinese women when dealing with potential psychiatric problems. Using a vignette depicting a major depression in a Chinese married woman, she interviewed a group of Chinese immigrant women at a San Francisco health center to explore the relationship between problem conceptualization and help-seeking behavior. When presented with the vignette, most women who conceptualized the problem as psychological did not suggest seeking professional psychological help; rather, they urged turning to family and friends or trying to resolve the problems themselves. On the other hand, those who conceptualized the problem as physical recommended seeking medical services.

Although data from other primary care providers serving Asian patients are not available, the impression of the community-based Asian health care providers is that many immigrant women, as well as men, are experiencing the strains of adapting to and surviving in a culturally divergent society and are expressing these strains as somatic complaints.

An explanation for this pattern is the significant cultural stigma attached to mental illness in most Asian countries; asking for help for somatic symptoms, however, is culturally acceptable. Compounding this cultural stigma, mental health services in Asian countries are designed to help the most seriously mentally ill. For this reason, those with moderate or less severe symptoms find it inconceivable to go to professionals for fear they might be considered "crazy." Under these circumstances, it will be important for mental health professionals to collaborate with primary care providers and provide consultation and training to improve their ability to deal with psychosomatic problems and to know when to make appropriate referrals to mental health providers.

Substance Abuse Problems. Although data on drug and alcohol abuse for the A/PI group are extremely limited, preliminary information includes data on gender differences. Several studies on the alcohol consumption patterns among Chinese, Japanese, Korean, Filipino, and Vietnamese Americans (Chi, Lubben, & Kitano, 1989; Padilla, Sung, & Nam, 1993) found that Asian American women were generally moderate or nondrinkers. Their low rate of drinking behavior is thought to be based on the strong cultural sanction in most Asian cultures against drinking by women. However, the pattern may be changing. For example, research conducted in Japan (Kono, Saito, Shimada, & Nakagawa, 1977) indicated a dramatic increase in the rate of women who drink, from 13% in 1954 to 53% in 1964.

Chi et al.'s (1989) survey of Asian Americans in the Los Angeles area revealed that Japanese women had the highest rate of heavy drinkers, 11.7%, and the lowest rate of abstainers, 33.4%; comparable rates for Chinese were 0% and 68.8%, for Koreans, .8% and 81.6%, and for Filipinos, 3.5% and 80.0%. Some contributing factors for these changes may be the impact of social changes, including blurring of sex roles, greater freedom for women, greater prosperity, and increased psychosocial stresses. The impact of acculturation is another factor to be considered for those living in the United States, as it was identified as the key factor for the changes in drinking patterns among Mexican American women (Markides, Ray, Stroup-Bebham, & Trevino, 1990).

The information on the use or abuse of drugs among A/PI women is even more limited, with conflicting findings. For example, Nakagawa and Watanabe (1973) interviewed Asian junior and senior high school students in Seattle and found that the use of hard drugs, excluding marijuana and alcohol, was considerable: 17% of female and 12% of male students were identified as users. Although gender differences were not cited, the differences between ethnic groups were significant in that 45% of the Filipino, 29% of the Japanese, and 22% of the Chinese students had some experience with hard drugs, including amphetamines, barbiturates, psychedelics, cocaine, and heroin (in descending order of frequency of use). However, more recent data from national surveys of high school seniors between 1976 and 1989 (Backman et al., 1991) indicate that the rates for Asian American females were significantly lower than those for white or Native American females for use of cigarettes, alcohol, and illicit drugs. Because information about country of origin or length of stay in the United States was not available, the question remains if acculturation is a factor in the increased rates of substance use for Asian American females.

Domestic Violence

Although data available on the extent of domestic violence against A/PI women are limited, many social service and women's shelter providers are concerned about the increasing incidence of abuse in A/PI communities in various parts of the country (Ho, 1990; Rimonte, 1989). They are particularly concerned about a possibly greater risk among more recently arrived A/PI immigrant and refugee women. A major contributing factor appears to be the significant level of frustration experienced by their male counterparts as they try unsuccessfully to establish themselves in the new country and find ways of supporting their families. In spite of their desire and effort, many of them have difficulty with English and do not have job skills that are transferrable and marketable in the United States.

On the other hand, women can find many jobs, although they are poorly paid, in domestic or other unskilled work; U.S.-born women are not willing to accept such work. When A/PI husbands are unable to find work or unable to support their families with marginal income, many women who did not work before immigration choose to get jobs to help support the family. In such situations, their husbands often feel humiliated, as if their masculinity or their authority as the patriarchal family head were damaged by having to rely on wives to support their families. At the same time, some wives become more assertive, feeling that with their greater role in supporting the family, they can expect to share decision-making authority on family matters. These changes in marital roles and relationship dynamics could often lead to considerable marital strife. Unaccustomed to such changes, some husbands take out their sense of powerlessness, rage, and frustration by abusing their wives, or they find escape in use of alcohol or drugs, which often leads to aggression against wives or children (Masaki, 1992; Rimonte, 1989).

Many abused A/PI women are reluctant to seek outside help, partly because of feelings of shame, fear of greater reprisals from abusers, and a sense of powerlessness. When they finally seek outside help, their plights are often ignored by service providers who do not understand the severity of the situation and are not sympathetic. Most appalling is when those with authority to intervene fail to do so and justify their nonaction by citing the need to respect Asian cultural tradition, which they believe condones oppression and violence against women. The case of a New York probation officer who recommended probation for a Chinese immigrant husband who murdered his wife, and the judge who accepted his recommendation, is the most galling instance of a failing system that ignores the plight of A/PI women (Hurtado, 1989). The argument used to justify such a light sentence for a heinous crime was based on their judgment that such an act was culturally acceptable in the family's native country (China) and that the husband was unlikely to commit other violent acts in the future (Hurtado, 1989). However, China has already made significant changes in recent years to protect the rights of women, establishing appropriate standards for punishment. Although acts of physical violence against women and wives still occur with some frequency and are overlooked in a few Asian countries, women advocates are

Table 7.1 Whites, Chinese, and Japanese: Average Annual Death Rates for Suicide, United States, 1980

| | Deaths per 100,000 Population | | | | | |
| | White | | Chinese | | Japanese | |
Age Group	Male	Female	Male	Female	Male	Female
All ages, crude	20.57	6.43	8.26	8.28	12.57	6.14
Age-adjusted	19.41	6.20	7.93	8.08	11.08	5.00
5-14 years	0.75	0.28		0.61	1.69	
15-24 years	21.91	5.00	8.07	4.65	14.09	4.52
25-34 years	26.99	7.98	8.59	5.72	16.72	7.82
35-44 years	24.27	9.93	8.94	9.09	12.68	6.39
45-54 years	24.55	11.18	10.77	13.89	9.81	8.22
55-64 years	26.52	9.59	9.37	15.52	12.38	7.78
65-74 years	32.41	7.45	25.85	22.61	11.17	2.17
75-84 years	46.18	6.03	21.82	44.32	39.56	15.75
85 years +	53.28	4.92	64.10	49.93	139.76	19.50

SOURCE: U.S. Department of Health and Human Services (1986, p. 26).
NOTE: In calculating age-specific death rates, the numerator consisted of 1979-1981 cumulative number of deaths and the denominator was based on the total enumerated in the 1981 U.S. census.

increasingly challenging the oppressive conditions in their countries (Sunda, 1994). Regardless of the conditions in Asia, A/PI women in the United States should be accorded the same protections as other American women and not be subjected to the abusive treatment that may still exist in other countries.

Suicides

Although suicide rates for combined age categories for A/PI Americans is low, some of the age and ethnicity subgroups are at higher risk than others, data indicate. For example, Yu and Liu (1986) analyzed the existing suicide data on Chinese and Japanese Americans and found that the rate for Chinese women increased dramatically beginning at ages 45 to 54; that rate was 15.52 per 100,000, increasing to 44.32 at ages 75 to 84 and 49.93 at ages 85 and over. In contrast, the rates for white women successively declined across the same age categories, beginning with a high of 11.18 at ages 45 to 54 (see Table 7.1).

Some of the stress factors that may be increasing suicide among elderly A/PI women include death of spouses whom they depended on for dealing with the English-speaking world, economic hardships, deteriorating health, decreasing support from their adult children, and the breakdown of extended family support networks. Although traditional A/PI cultures place a strong value on treating elders with respect and care, immigrant families are separated from the extended family network and have limited resources to care for aging parents. Some families have to live and work in areas far away from their parents so that it is not possible for them to provide day-to-day support.

The number of A/PI people over 65 years of age is projected to increase dramatically, from 450,000 to 2.1 million by 2020, representing a 355% increase (Ong & Hee, 1992), and A/PI women, like women in general, tend to live longer than men. Thus, they will likely continue to experience significant stresses from poverty, isolation, lack of support, and declining health and be at risk for suicide.

Psychosocial Stressors

Many sources of stress contribute to the development of mental health problems for A/PI women. Foremost among these are those related to immigration and acculturation. When they arrive in the United States, many immigrant women are confronted by an unfamiliar language, lifestyle changes, and day-to-day survival issues. Although many had to deal with survival issues in their old country, they were able to rely on a supportive extended family and community network for help; now they can no longer rely on this help. Although some are able to replace the lost support with new neighbors, many are unable to create another network, perhaps due to work or their traditional reluctance to seek help beyond the family kinship network (Bradshaw, 1994; True, 1991).

Immigrant women also experience significant conflict with their children, who become more rapidly acculturated and demand greater independence and freedom in making their own choices about friends, dating, sexuality, field of study, and occupation. Meanwhile, parents often become much more restrictive in an effort to shield children from what they perceive as negative influences in the outside community. Because of the old-world attitude toward women, parents are often more restrictive toward daughters, believing they need to work hard to protect them against "loose morals" so that they will not fall prey to such social ills as promiscuity, teenage pregnancy, and substance abuse. However, this, in turn, makes daughters resentful and rebellious: They know American girls are given much greater freedom than they have. The conflict is often most keenly felt between mothers and daughters, because mothers are expected to socialize their daughters to be compliant with the proper expectations for Asian women, that is, to be faithful to their parents, to be submissive to their men, and so on. Such struggles are poignantly portrayed in Amy Tan's (1989) book, *The Joy Luck Club*, and have been described by mental health professionals working with adolescent girls who struggle not only with their parents at home but with a variety of adjustment problems at schools (Kope & Sack, 1987; Williams & Westermeyer, 1983).

Native-born Asian American women and others who are freer of the basic survival needs faced by immigrant women face different types of stresses. Frequently, they are subjected to the double jeopardy of discrimination in various social and work settings because of their status as members of racial and sexual minority groups. Whatever their own individual strengths and abilities, A/PI women are often treated according to stereotypes that have a negative impact on them. For example, because the media often portray them as sexually promiscuous and easily accommodating, in such roles as Suzy Wong and Miss Saigon, they may be perceived as sex objects to be exploited. They are also often considered to be subservient, passive handmaidens or weak, helpless, dependent women who will be good office helpers, but who do not possess much leadership quality in work settings and are not deserving of promotional opportunities. If an A/PI woman is somewhat aggressive, she is quickly typecast as a power-hungry, ruthless "dragon lady."

A/PI women also experience difficulties within their own families and communities, where they are often treated as inferior to men in status and are expected to sacrifice their own personal needs to the needs of their men. This is a legacy of traditional, patriarchal Asian cultures, where women were oppressed for centuries and were expected to be subservient to males in all stages of their lives. It is generally assumed that older Asian women, particularly those who were born abroad and have had limited exposure to the more liberal Western perception of women's status and roles, are more accepting or resigned to this cultural expectation (True, 1991).

However, many younger women are dissatisfied with the traditional expectations imposed on them as second-class citizens in their community. Increasing numbers of these women now have the opportunity to seek higher education and are exposed to the radically different treatment of women in the larger American community. During the period when university campuses throughout the United States were activated by the civil rights movement, many A/PI women students became involved in campus activities and had their consciousness raised by the feminist movement (Chow, 1989; Fujitomi & Wong, 1973). Although initially apprehensive about the potential conflict of feminist ideologies and minority concerns related to the experience of racism, many younger A/PI women are now convinced that they need to challenge the pervasive stereotypes and discriminatory treatment of their counterparts, and they are struggling to define their new identity so that they can take pride in their individuality and be accepted by others on equal terms.

Another recent trend emerging as potential source of strain for A/PI women is the increasing number of interethnic and interracial marriages. Although interracial marriages were strongly discouraged in the United States by both Asian and mainstream communities, as well as antimiscegenation legislation in the early years of Asian immigration, it is begrudgingly recognized now as a trend that will grow in the future (Kikumura & Kitano, 1973; Shinagawa & Pang, 1988). When young people are first swept away by romantic love, many do not realize the potential conflicts associated with the fact they grew up with divergent cultural backgrounds, values, beliefs, and so on, and are ill-prepared to deal with these differences (Ho, 1990). This is particularly true for partners with widely divergent backgrounds, such as those involving the so-called war brides from Asian countries where U.S. servicemen were stationed (Kim, 1977) or more recent "mail-order brides," who are being brought in through advertisements from Asian countries. Although U.S.-born A/PI women who outmarry do not suffer from language problems and share more cultural experiences with their partners than their foreign-born counterparts, they also find themselves confronted with relationship problems they did not anticipate, often rooted in cultural differences. In addition to the strains due to cultural differences, both Asian-born and U.S.-born women are often subjected to racist hostilities from others because of long-standing social prejudices against intermarriage.

The challenges faced by biracial or multiracial Asian women, the offspring of these marriages, are also complex. Those who are more vulnerable will face additional strains, but the multicultural environment can also provide rich opportunities for personal growth for those who are willing or able to embrace the challenges (Root, 1992).

Service Strategies

Most service providers working with A/PI women received their training in U.S. educational institutions and use a variety of psychotherapeutic approaches based on Western conceptual and theoretical orientations. These include a variety of psychodynamic approaches, cognitive therapy, behavioral therapy, and various family therapy approaches. Although more Westernized A/PI women can benefit from application of these treatment approaches, many service providers have learned that considerable adjustment is needed for services to many A/PI women (Bradshaw, 1994; Shon & Ja, 1982; Sue & Morishima, 1982; Tien, 1994; True, 1990).

Some key elements of effective service strategies for A/PI individuals in general also apply to A/PI women. They include the following:

Availability of bilingual, bicultural therapists for non-English speaking clients. It is critical that every effort be made to make bilingual and bicultural mental health providers available to non-English speaking clients. In their guidelines for working with ethnic, linguistic, and culturally diverse populations, the American Psychological Association (1991) acknowledges the need for competent interpreters or translators in the absence of bilingual, bicultural professionals, but it also cautions about the limitations and risk of reliance on interpreters.

Location of services within geographically accessible locations and flexible hours. Many immigrant women are not only fearful of approaching a mental health program because of the cultural stigma, but they have a great deal of difficulty traveling outside of their communities to an impersonal institution.

Collaboration with primary care clinics and providers to deal with the tendency somatize psychological distress. As demonstrated by Yu et al. (1987) and Ying (1990), many A/PI women are more receptive to receiving help in the early stages of difficulties at primary care health service sites, and efforts should be made to collaborate with these service providers.

Multiservice approach. Discussing mental health services for work with minority women, Olmedo and Parron (1981) advocated linking psychotherapy with education, health, and social services on the basis that this approach can address not only the immediate mental health problems, but also the environmental, economic, and social factors that affect the mental health of minority women. Such an approach is particularly helpful with Asian American women, whose mental health problems are often directly related to adverse financial and social problems.

Involvement of families. Because A/PI groups are strongly family-oriented, it is important, when working with individual clients, to consider the interrelationship between them and family members. Often, it is important to involve parents, spouses, and other family members in working with individual clients. When talking about the need for a family-focused approach, many of the Asian therapists also stress the need to respect the traditional patriarchal family structure (Shon & Ja, 1982). Particular attention is paid to the role of the husband and father as the key decision maker in the family. This is followed by the need to respect the parents as part of filial obligations. However, others are beginning to raise concerns about the need to balance family integrity and the degree to which a woman's own personal needs should be sacrificed. For Asian women, the personal cost of accepting the stressful family status quo could eventually lead to serious psychiatric difficulties. When domestic violence is involved, failure to intervene could lead to tragic consequences.

Sensitivity to women's unique needs and problems. Much has been written about sex role stereotyping and treatment bias of practicing U.S. therapists toward female patients. Many concerned female mental health professionals have pioneered the development of treatment approaches and advocated for the efficacy of gender matches for certain types of female patients (Mowbray & Benedek, 1988). Because of the pervasive sexism toward A/PI women, they are also often given inappropriate treatment that does not resolve the destructive status quo. In this respect, A/PI women therapists, who are more sensitized about the plight of their counterparts, can be helpful in advocating for their needs (True, 1990). A review of Los Angeles County data at the National Research Center for Asian American Mental Health (Sue, Fujino, Hu, Takeuchi, & Zane, 1991) also seems to suggest that gender match was helpful for Asian American clients in lowering dropout rates and achieving better treatment outcomes.

Conclusion and Recommendations

Despite a lack of specific data about the mental health status or service use of A/PI women, indications are that they experience considerable stress. Some factors affecting their mental health status were identified as stresses related to their pre- and postimmigration strains, acculturation conflict, marital and family conflict, and various experiences of racism and sexism. In spite of the problems they are experiencing, however, A/PI women are reluctant to seek professional mental health services. The factors influencing their service underuse were identified as partly due to the cultural stigma within their communities. Other factors include unavailability of bilingual, bicultural service providers, fears about institutional agencies, and the problem of accessibility due to geographic location and available hours. Creative approaches could reverse this situation.

As the number of A/PI women is growing rapidly, their problems are also expected to increase. It is critical that greater attention and support be provided to identify and address their mental health issues. The following are some of the actions needed to improve this situation:

- Funding and technical support is needed for research focused on the mental health needs of Asian Pacific American women, for example, epidemiology, psychosocial stressors, and risk factors, with provisions for identifying subgroup and regional differences.
- Aggressive recruitment and support should be provided for training of A/PI mental health professionals to develop expertise on A/PI women's issues, as well as linguistic, bicultural capacity.
- Both non-A/PI professionals and A/PI male professionals need training to increase their cultural sensitivity toward A/PI women's needs.
- There should be increased funding to develop linguistically and culturally appropriate services for A/PI women, including outreach and education.
- Provision of ancillary services, such as social services, child care, vocational training, housing, and homemaker services to high-risk populations is needed to reduce the level of psychosocial stresses that often lead to the development of psychiatric and psychological difficulties.

References

American Psychological Association. (1991). *Guidelines for providers of psychological services to ethnic, linguistic, and culturally diverse population.* Washington, DC: Author.

Backman, J. G., Wallace, J. M., O'Malley, P. M., Johnston, L. D., Kurth, C. L., & Neighbors, H. W. (1991). Racial/ethnic differences in smoking, drinking, and illicit drug use among American high school seniors, 1976-1989. *American Journal of Public Health, 81*(3), 372-377.

Bradshaw, C. K. (1994). Asian and Asian American women: Historical and political considerations in psychotherapy. In L. Comas-Diaz & B. Greene (Eds.), *Women of color: Integrating ethnic and gender identities in psychotherapy* (pp. 72-113). New York: Guilford.

California Department of Mental Health. (1992). *Local mental health programs: Unduplicated clients served fiscal year 1989-90.* Sacramento, CA: Author.

Chi, I., Lubben, J. D., & Kitano, H. H. L. (1989). Differences in drinking behavior among three Asian American groups. *Journal of Studies on Alcohol, 50*(1), 15-23.

Chow, E. N.-L. (1989). The feminist movement: Where are all the Asian American women. In Asian Women United of California (Ed.), *Making waves: An anthology of writings by and about Asian-American women* (pp. 362-377). Boston: Beacon Press.

Chung, R. C. (1991, August). *Predictors of distress among Southeast Asian refugees: Group and gender differences.* Paper presented at Asian American Psychological Association Conference, San Francisco.

Fujino, D. C., & Chung, R. C. (1991, August). *Asian American mental health: An examination of gender issues.* Paper presented at the annual convention of Asian American Psychological Association, San Francisco.

Fujitomi, I., & Wong, D. (1973). The new Asian American women. In S. Sue & N. Wagner (Eds.), *Asian Americans: Psychological perspectives.* (pp. 252-263). Palo Alto, CA: Science and Behavior Books.

Gong-Guy, E. (1987). *The California Southeast Asian mental health needs assessment.* Oakland, CA: Asian Community Mental Health Services.

Ho, C. (1990). An analysis of domestic violence in Asian American communities. *Women and Therapy, 9*(1-2), 129-150.

Hurh, W. M., & Kim, K. C. (1990). Correlates of Korean immigrants' mental health. *Journal of Nervous and Mental Disorder, 178*(11), 703-711.

Hurtado, P. (1989, April 4). Killer's sentence defended: "He's not a loose cannon." *Newsday,* pp. 3, 25.

Jayakar, K. (1994). Women of the Indian subcontinent. In L. Comas-Diaz & B. Greene (Eds.), *Women of color: Integrating ethnic and gender identities in psychotherapy* (pp. 161-184). New York: Guilford.

Kikumura, A., & Kitano, H. (1973). Interracial marriage: A picture of the Japanese Americans. *Journal of Social Issues, 29*(2), 67-81.

Kim, B.-L. C. (1977). Asian wives of U.S. servicemen: Women in shadows. *Amerasia, 4,* 91-115.

Kono, H. , Saito, S., Shimada, K., & Nakagawa, J. (1977). *Drinking habits of the Japanese.* Tokyo: Leisure Development Center.

Kope, T. M., & Sack, W. H. (1987). Anorexia nervosa in Southeast Asian refugees: A report on three cases. *Journal of American Academy of Child and Adolescent Psychiatry, 26*(5), 794-797.

Lee, I. S. (Ed.). (1985). *Korean American women: Toward self-realization.* Mansfield, OH: Association of Korean Christian Scholars in Northern America.

Lin, T. Y., Rin, H., Yeh, E., Hsu, C., & Chu, H. (1969). Mental disorder in Taiwan, fifteen years later: A preliminary report. In W. Caudill & T. Y. Liu (Eds.), *Mental health research in Asia and the Pacific* (pp. 66-91). Honolulu: East-West Press.

Markides, K., Ray, L., Stroup-Bebham, C., & Trevino, F. (1990). Acculturation and alcohol consumption in the Mexican American population of the Southwestern United States: Findings from HHANES, 1982-84. *American Journal of Public Health, 80,* 42-46.

Masaki, B. (1992). Shattered myths: Battered women in the A/PI community. *Focus, 3,* 1, 3.

Mowbray, C. T., & Benedek, E. P. (1988). *Women's mental health research agenda: Services and treatment of mental disorders in women* (Women's Mental Health Occasional Paper Series). Rockville, MD: National Institute of Mental Health.

Nagata, D. (1991). Transgenerational impact of the Japanese-American internment: Clinical issues in working with children of former internees. *Psychotherapy, 28*(1), 121-128.

Nakagawa, B., & Watanabe, R. (1973). *A study of the use of drugs among Asian American youths of Seattle.* Seattle: Demonstration Project for Asian Americans.

Nakano, M. (1990). *Japanese American women: Three generations 1890-1990.* Berkeley: MINA Press.

Navarro, J. (1976). Immigration of Filipino women to America. In *Asian American women* (pp. 18-22). Stanford, CA: Asian American Studies, Stanford University.

Olmedo, E. L., & Parron, D. L. (1981). Mental health of minority women: Some special issues. *Professional Psychology, 12*(1), 103-111.

Ong, P., & Hee, S. J. (1992). The growth of the Asian Pacific American population: Twenty million in 2020. In LEAP Asian Pacific American Public Policy Institute and UCLA Asian American Studies Center (Eds.), *The state of Asian Pacific America: Policy Issues to the year 2020* (pp. 11-24). Los Angeles: LEAP Asian Pacific American Public Policy Institute and UCLA Asian American Studies Center.

Padilla, A., Sung, H., & Nam, T. V. (1993, Winter). Attitudes toward alcohol and drinking practices in two Vietnamese samples in Santa Clara County. *Horizons of Vietnamese Thought and Experience, 2*(1), 53-71.

President's Commission on Mental Health. (1978). *Report to the president: Volume 4.* Washington, DC: Government Printing Office.

Radloff, L. S. (1977). The CES-D scale: A self-report depression scale for research in the general population. *Applied Psychological Measurement, 1,* 385-401.

Rimonte, N. (1989). Domestic violence among Pacific Asians. In Asian Women United of California (Ed.), *Making waves: An anthology of writings by and about Asian American women* (pp. 327-336). Boston: Beacon Press.

Robbins, L. N., Locke, B., & Regier, D. A. (1991). An overview of psychiatric disorders in America. In L. N. Robbins & D. A. Regier (Eds.), *Psychiatric disorders in America: The Epidemiologic Catchment Area study* (p. 350). New York: Free Press.

Rozee, P. D., & Van Boemel, G. (1989). The psychological effects of war trauma and abuse on older Cambodian refugee women. *Women and Therapy, 8*(4), 23-49.

Rumbaut, R. G. (1985). Mental health and the refugee experience: A comparative study of Southeast Asian refugees. In T. C. Owan (Ed.), *Southeast Asian mental health: Treatment, prevention, services, training, and research* (pp. 433-486). Washington, DC: National Institute of Mental Health.

Shinagawa, L. H., & Pang, G. Y. (1988). Intraethnic, interethnic, and interracial marriages among Asian Americans in California. *Berkeley Journal of Sociology, 33,* 95-114.

Shon, S. P., & Ja, D. Y. (1982). Asian families. In M. McGodrick, J. K. Pearce, & J. Giordano (Eds.), *Ethnicity and family therapy* (pp. 208-228). New York: Guilford.

Snowden, L. R., & Cheung, F. K. (1990). Use of inpatient mental health services by members of ethnic minority groups. *American Psychologist, 45,* 347-355.

Sue, S. (1988). Psychotherapeutic services for ethnic minorities: Two decades of research findings. *American Psychologist, 43,* 301-308.

Sue, S., Fujino, D. C., Hu, L., Takeuchi, D. T., & Zane, N. W. S. (1991). Community mental health services for ethnic minority groups: A test of the cultural responsiveness hypothesis. *Journal of Clinical and Consulting Psychology, 59*(4), 533-540.

Sue, S., & McKinney, H. (1975). Asian Americans in the community mental health care system. *American Journal of Orthopsychiatry, 45,* 11-18.

Sue, S., & Morishima, J. K. (1982). *The mental health of Asian Americans.* San Francisco: Jossey-Bass.

Sunda, M. (1994). India: Rethinking sex crimes. *Ms., 4,* 5, 20.

Takaki, R. (1989). *Strangers from a different shore: History of Asian Americans.* Boston: Little, Brown.

Tan, A. (1989). *The joy luck club*. New York: Ballantine.

Tien, L. (1994). Southeast Asian American refugee women. In L. Comas-Diaz & B. Greene (Eds.), *Women of color: Integrating ethnic and gender identities in psychotherapy* (pp. 479-504). New York: Guilford.

True, R. H. (1990). Psychotherapeutic issues with Asian American women. *Sex Roles, 22*(7/8), 477-486.

True, R. H. (1991, August). *Psychosocial impact of immigration on Asian women*. Paper presented at the annual convention of American Psychological Association, San Francisco.

U.S. Bureau of the Census. (1992, August). The Asian and Pacific Islander population in the United States: March 1991 and 1990. In *Current population reports* (pp. 20-459). Washington, DC: Government Printing Office.

U.S. Bureau of the Census. (1993). *We, the American . . . Asians*. Washington, DC: Government Printing Office.

U.S. Department of Health and Human Services (1986). *Report of the Secretary's Task Force on Black and Minority Health: Vol. 5. Homicide, suicide, and unintentional injuries*. Washington, DC: Author.

Williams, C. L., & Westermeyer, J. (1983). Psychiatric problems among adolescent Southeast Asian refugees. *Journal of Nervous and Mental Disease, 171*(2), 79-85.

Ying, Y. W. (1988). Depressive symptomatology among Chinese-Americans as measured by the CES-D. *Journal of Clinical Psychology, 44*(5), 739-746.

Ying, Y. W. (1990). Explanatory models of major depression and implications for help-seeking among immigrant Chinese-American women. *Culture, Medicine, and Psychiatry, 14*, 393-408.

Yu, E. S. H., & Liu, W. T. (1986). Whites, Chinese, and Japanese: Average annual death rates for suicide, United States, 1980. In *Report of the Secretary's Task Force on Black and Minority Health: Vol. 5. Homicide, suicide, and unintentional injuries* (p. 26). Washington, DC: U.S. Department of Health and Human Services.

Yu, E. S. H., Liu, W. T., & Wong, S. C. (1987). Measurement of depression in a Chinatown health clinic. In W. T. Liu (Ed.), *A decade review of mental health research, training, and services* (pp. 95-100). Chicago: Pacific/Asian American Mental Health Research Center, University of Illinois at Chicago.

Yung, J. (1986). *Chinese women of America: A pictorial history*. Seattle: University of Washington Press.

8 The Health of African American Women

WILHELMINA A. LEIGH

In 1991, over half (16.4 million) of the more than 31 million African Americans were females (U.S. Bureau of the Census, 1993). African American or Black American females, like all women, receive health care in the context of the families in which they perform multiple caregiving roles—as wives, mothers, daughters, widows, single childless women, and so on. These caregiving roles often translate into interrupted employment histories and limited access to health insurance, and they place time constraints on women's ability to seek care for themselves. Dependence on a husband for health insurance coverage leaves the caregiver wife vulnerable if the marriage dissolves or if the employer cuts back on or eliminates dependent coverage.

These general problems and characteristics of women as caregivers and consumers of health care services are compounded for African American women by the special circumstances of their lives and the lives of the men about whom they care. Prejudice, discrimination,

AUTHOR'S NOTE: This analysis is the author's own and should not be attributed to the Joint Center for Political and Economic Studies, its board of governors, or its sponsors.

112

and poverty all interact to generate the daily diet of stresses that bear on their health.

This chapter provides information on the health of African American women. The first section, which borrows heavily from other work done by the author, establishes the context for the health of African Americans (Leigh, 1994a). The second section discusses health habits and lifestyles, and the third describes access to health insurance and health care services. The fourth section covers the incidence of disease and mortality for both African American and White women. The fifth section raises issues related to health care reform, and the final section provides conclusions for the chapter.

Context

Differences in the health of Blacks and Whites are many and varied. Blacks have more undetected diseases, higher disease and illness rates, and more chronic conditions (such as hypertension and diabetes) than Whites (Leffall, 1990). Mortality rates for Blacks from many conditions (cancer, HIV/AIDS, and homicide) exceed those for Whites. Explanations for these racial differences have been sought by experts, and many contributing factors have been identified. The major factors—genetics, poverty, and racism—are discussed below.

The murkiness of race as a concept to define Black Americans, who range from fair-skinned and blue-eyed to dark-skinned with coarse hair, makes purely genetic explanations of the health differences between Blacks and Whites questionable. Biology appears to explain very few of the differences in health between Blacks and Whites, if the proportion of excess deaths among Blacks—that is, deaths that would not have occurred if Blacks experienced the same age- and sex-related death rates as Whites—due to hereditary conditions is examined. Less than 1% of Black deaths have been attributed to hereditary conditions such as sickle cell anemia, for which genetic patterns have been established (Jaynes & Williams, 1989). On the other hand, researchers studying the incidence of hypertension among Blacks have found that it varies with skin color. That is, lighter-pigmented Blacks have a lower prevalence of hypertension than darker-skinned Blacks, and pigment is related to the degree of admixture with Whites, whose overall incidence of hypertension is lower than that of Blacks (Wilkinson & King, 1989).

Instead of looking at population-related genetic differences, others link the racial differences in health to Black subpopulations that are exposed to multiple risks, such as intravenous drug users, those living and working in hazardous environments, and the like. Health conditions common among Blacks that are considered to be genetic in origin are likely to receive more public attention and resources than conditions that arise from behavior or lifestyle choices. For example, conditions such as sickle cell anemia receive more research attention and public support than health conditions attributable to accidents, substance abuse, and environmentally caused illnesses (Wilkinson & King, 1989).

Poverty affected nearly one third of all Black Americans (31.9%) and 35.5% of all Black women in 1990. Single-parent, female-headed households, 44% of all Black households in 1990, were mired in poverty to a greater degree than the entire Black population (U.S. Bureau of the Census, 1992c). About 48% of all Black female-headed families had incomes below the poverty level in 1990, and 75% of the 2 million Black families in poverty were maintained by women with no husbands present (U.S. Bureau of the Census, 1992a).

Inadequate income carries over into other aspects of daily life that impinge upon health. These include inadequate housing (with its risk of injury and illnesses such as lead poisoning), malnutrition, the stress of constantly struggling to make ends meet, dangerous jobs, and little or no preventive medical care. Malnutrition in Black girls may result in low birth weight babies and high infant mortality rates when these girls become mothers. The stresses of constantly struggling to make ends meet may translate directly into the finding that Blacks below the poverty level have the highest rate of depression for any group (Liu & Yu, 1985). Dangerous jobs (and living environments) may expose Blacks to certain cancers to a much greater extent than Whites (Miller, 1989).

According to Headen and Headen (1985-1986) and Jaynes and Williams (1989), little or no preventive care may come about for a variety of reasons, including

parental ignorance of disease symptoms and when to seek medical care;
lack of health insurance to enable access to health care;

lack of neighborhood facilities in which to seek health care;

persistent use of emergency rooms to treat chronic conditions, which are better managed in other settings; and

racial discrimination encountered when seeking care.

Racial discrimination and racism have remained significant operative factors in the health status and health care of Blacks over time. From as early as 1867, Black experts concluded that racism was a major contributor to the poor health of Black Americans in two significant ways. First, *structural racism* creates barriers to getting access to adequate care, and second, dealing with both structural barriers and racial insults may contribute to stress-related health problems, such as pregnancy-induced hypertension among Black women (Hogue & Hargraves, 1993).

John Henryism, defined as the behavioral predisposition to work hard and strive determinedly against the constraints of one's environment, has been advanced as an explanation for the Black-White differences in hypertension rates. High blood pressure in Blacks is a response to the incongruity between the social position one's work would typically merit and the position one actually occupies (Smith & Egger, 1992).

Racial discrimination has limited the access of Blacks to higher incomes, improved health care, adequate housing, and better education—all of which are necessary to achieve modern levels of health and mortality (Ewbank, 1989). Racial discrimination probably "exacerbates the mental health-damaging effects of poverty status among Blacks" (Miller, 1989, p. 511). Being Black impinges upon health, even at higher income levels. A study of stress found its severity highest in lower-class Blacks and lowest in middle-class Whites. Even more notable is the fact that middle-class Blacks and lower-class Whites had similar levels of stress (Miller, 1989).

Another example of what may be a physiological response to racism is pregnancy outcome. Mortality rates for infants born to college-educated Black parents (from 1983 to 1985) were 90% higher than the rates among infants born to college-educated White parents. This excess mortality was due primarily to higher rates of death associated with premature delivery of Black babies (Schoendorf, Hogue, Kleinman, & Rowley, 1992). In addition, immigrant Black couples have a lower incidence of low birth weight babies than native-born Black couples. The incidence of low birth weight babies among immigrant Blacks is similar to the incidence among White couples. Moreover, Black babies born in more segregated cities have higher rates of infant mortality than their counterparts born in less segregated cities (Hogue & Hargraves, 1993).

The impact on health of responses to racism also can be seen by the high mortality rates for Blacks from cancer and HIV/AIDS. Blacks are both less educated about the danger signs for cancer and more pessimistic about treatment for cancer than are Whites. Both of these facts interact to make cancer the terminal disease Blacks conceive it to be (Manton, Patrick, & Johnson, 1989).

It has been suggested that the experience of fighting HIV/AIDS is different for most Whites than for minorities and the poor. For Whites with HIV/AIDS, the fact that they have education and employment contributes to their sense of outrage about the disease and motivates them to fight for what is being lost. Blacks and members of other minority groups, who may never have had these advantages, do not have this sense of loss, the associated drive to fight against the loss, and the educational tools with which to wage the fight. Delays in seeking medical care, differences in preexisting health, and differences in drugs administered as treatment generate a mean survival time of 6 months for Blacks after diagnosis with HIV/AIDS, whereas Whites have a mean survival time of 18 to 24 months (Friedman et al., 1989).

Resentment of others at the unfair advantages presumably accorded Blacks under affirmative action programs contributes to the sense of exclusion from and inequality in mainstream America felt by Blacks, a sense that affects them economically, socially, and physically. Even if poverty in America is reduced, as long as economic, social, and political inequalities persist, the health of Black Americans is likely to remain impaired (Miller, 1989).

Health Habits and Lifestyles

Lifestyle patterns influence the health and incidence of disease in all Americans. Among these are overeating (which can lead to obesity and high serum cholesterol) and abusing substances. These lifestyle patterns, along with selected preventive measures or health habits, are discussed in the next sections.

OBESITY AND HIGH SERUM CHOLESTEROL

A condition associated with diabetes, hypertension, and cardio-vascular disease, obesity is a problem for African American women and is related in part to the "diets of poverty"—high in fat and low in fruits and vegetables—that many of these women consume. Defined as excess body weight for height, or being overweight, obesity affects 50% of Black women between the ages of 20 and 74, and 34% of their White age and gender peers, based on data from 1988 to 1991 (National Center for Health Statistics [NCHS], 1995).

High serum cholesterol—a factor in cardiovascular disease often found in conjunction with obesity—is a problem for White women 20 to 74 years of age nearly as often as for African American women in that age group. About 20% of White women and 21% of Black women were reported to have high serum cholesterol, in surveys conducted between 1988 and 1991 (NCHS, 1995).

Although obesity is more of a problem for Black women than for White women, and high cholesterol levels seem to be found equally among the two groups, some of the factors associated with overeating differ for the two groups. Overeating is a common response to stress for all people. For some Black women and men (and for other disadvantaged groups in U.S. society), stress is compounded by the pervasive psychological effects of racism to generate chronic obesity. In addition, the quality and type of food—that is, low or high in fat—consumed is influenced by what is readily available. A majority of all Black Americans—60%—live in America's central cities, in neighborhoods that are often bereft of supermarkets (Leigh, 1994b). Reliance on "mom-and-pop" stores for food, because poverty and other health infirmities make it difficult to leave the immediate environs to do grocery shopping, limits many Black women to a diet of high calorie/low fiber foods.

Other factors in obesity among Black women are their attitudes toward body size and dieting and how these differ from the attitudes of White women. In a sample of women aged 66 to 105 years, over-weight Black women were less likely to feel guilty after overeating and less likely to diet than were overweight White women. Overweight Black women also were more likely to be satisfied with their weight (2.5 times as often as overweight White women) and more likely to consider themselves attractive (2.5 times as likely as overweight White women) (Stevens, Kumanyika, & Keil, 1994). These differences in attitudes suggest differences in the motivation to lose weight for Black and White women that may contribute to the obesity disparity reported.

SUBSTANCE ABUSE

The major substances abused in the United States are cigarettes, alcohol, and illicit drugs, such as heroin, cocaine, and marijuana. When data for the use of these substances are examined, Black women are found to have lower propensity to report being current smokers, a lower propensity to report being current drinkers, and a greater propensity to report current use of any illicit drug.

Although the data differ slightly from survey to survey, if lifetime use of cigarettes is examined, 73% of White females report ever smoking whereas only 63% of Black females have ever smoked (Horton, 1992). Current cigarette smoking shows a different pattern. Although smoking has declined among both Black and White females since the late 1980s, 20% of Black and 24% of White females 18 years and older reported in 1993 that they currently smoked (NCHS, 1995).

Alcohol consumption becomes a factor in women's health if it is frequent and heavy enough to impair their judgment, to place women at risk of accidents and abuse by others, and to result in fetal damage among pregnant women. About 83% of White women and 75% of Black women have used alcohol at some point in their lives (Horton, 1992).

Black women (46%) are more likely to abstain from alcohol than are White women (34%), although equal proportions drink heavily (U.S. Department of Health & Human Services, n.d.). In 1990, about 38% of Black women 18 to 44 years of age reported that they were current drinkers, compared to 65% of White women. Although the figures were lower among women 45 years and older, the pattern was the same—a larger share of White women (44%) than of Black women (25%) in this age range reported that they were current drinkers (NCHS, 1995).

Both African American women and White women report having used illicit substances, risking their own health and that of their unborn children. Slightly more White women (35%) than Black women (33%) report using illicit drugs at some point in their lives. Current use of any illicit drug, however, is slightly higher among Black women (7%) than among White women (5%) (Horton, 1992). Use of any illicit drugs during pregnancy also is greater among Black than White women. About 11% of Black women and 4% of White women are estimated to have engaged in any illicit drug use during pregnancy (National Institute on Drug Abuse, 1994).

As with overeating, abusing substances is often associated with stress, depression, anxiety, trauma, and so on among the population in general. As noted above, stress and depression both have high incidence among African American women. Anxiety and trauma also are intertwined in the lives of African American women, as evidenced by the high homicide rates among African Americans. Although homicide and legal intervention were the cause of death for only 13 African American women per 100,000 in 1992, the rate for African American men was 68 per 100,000 (NCHS, 1995). Deaths of African American men affect the African American women who are their mates, wives, mothers, sisters, and so on, and for some of those women, these deaths are the precipitating factor in substance abuse.

Preventive Measures

African American women often do not avail themselves of preventive health tests such as Pap smears and breast examinations. For example, although the incidence of cervical cancer among Blacks is twice that among Whites, African American women underuse Pap smears and mammography. About 66% of Black women report that their last Pap smear was less than a year ago. About 78% of Black women in the 45 years and older age group report ever having had a mammogram (Communications Consortium, n.d). For never-married, childless African American women, the need to seek preventive services is as great as for wives and mothers. However, sometimes childless women neglect tests such as Pap smears and mammograms, thinking they are unnecessary, because they have never borne children. In fact, a study by Calle, Flanders, Thun, and

Martin (1993) found that never having been married was a strong predictor of never having a Pap smear.

Another preventive service that many believe contributes to the delivery of a healthy baby is prenatal care in the first trimester of pregnancy. In 1992, only 64% of Black mothers received early care, compared to nearly 81% of White mothers-to-be (NCHS, 1995). Women who receive late or no prenatal care were more likely to be poor, adolescent, unmarried, rural dwellers, or over 40 years of age—characteristics that place their pregnancies at high risk from other causes as well (Jaynes & Williams, 1989).

Access to Health Insurance and Health Care Services

Access to health care includes both access to health insurance coverage and access to providers and facilities that render services. Adequate access to providers and facilities encompasses the existence of conveniently located services and the availability of child care (to enable mothers to seek medical attention), transportation, and health care providers capable of giving sensitive and competent care.

OBTAINING HEALTH INSURANCE COVERAGE

Although wives are often insured as dependents of their husbands, estimates show that between 13% and 14% of all women, or 16 to 17 million women, lack insurance (Horton, 1992). Just as African Americans make up a sizable proportion of the uninsured—16% of the uninsured, although they comprise only 12% of the total population—African American women make up a sizable proportion of all uninsured women.

Lack of health insurance is a more severe problem for Blacks than for Whites, with Blacks 1.8 times as likely to be uninsured as Whites (Assocation of Asian Pacific Community Health Organizations, n.d.; Horton, 1992). In 1990, nearly 6.1 million Blacks (or about 20% of all Blacks) and 26.9 million Whites (or 12.9% of the entire White population) were uninsured (National Council of La Raza, 1992). Because of Medicare enrollment by the elderly the proportions uninsured were slightly higher for people under age 65—23% of Blacks and 16% of Whites (NCHS, 1995).

Blacks are also considerably less likely to have private health insurance (and the additional options and greater coverage it often affords) and are more likely to have public insurance than are Whites. In 1993, whereas 75% of Whites had private health insurance, more than half (51%) of Blacks did (Short et al., 1990). In addition, between February 1987 and May 1989, 40% of Blacks and 24% of Whites were without health insurance coverage for at least a month. Women were slightly less likely than men (25% versus 28%) to have had gaps in coverage for two reasons. First, it was more common for women to live in families with incomes below the poverty level and, therefore, to be eligible for and to be enrolled in Medicaid. Second, a higher percentage of women than men were over 65 years of age and were likely to be enrolled in Medicare (U.S. Bureau of the Census, 1992b).

Blacks also are heavily enrolled in public insurance (Medicaid, Medicare, and public coverage through the Department of Veterans Affairs and the military). About 26% of Blacks under 65 years of age had public insurance in 1987, and Blacks make up roughly 40% of all Medicaid enrollees (Rice & Winn, 1991; Short, Cornelius, & Goldstone, 1990). However, many Blacks reside in southern states where Medicaid benefits are the least generous. Although all states place constraints on enrollment and limits on health services, the southern states impose the most severe ones (Leffall, 1990). Many health care providers refuse to accept Medicaid reimbursement because it falls too far short of the costs incurred to provide services. Thus Blacks who receive coverage through Medicaid might more properly be called underinsured and be added to the estimated 1 to 2 million Black Americans whose health insurance coverage is inadequate for their needs (Jaynes & Williams, 1989).

OBTAINING HEALTH CARE SERVICES

One step beyond health insurance coverage is making contact with physicians or other providers. In the 1977 National Medical Care Expenditure Survey, the percentages of Blacks and Whites who stated that a physician's office was their usual source of care were 46% and 70%, respectively (Delgado & Treviño, 1985). In contrast, in 1993, 48%

of Blacks and 58% of Whites reported the physician's office as the usual place of contact for care. Blacks report the hospital outpatient department (including hospital outpatient clinic, emergency room, and other hospital contacts) as their usual place of physician contact more often than Whites (21% versus 12%) (NCHS, 1995).

There are many reasons why Blacks report using hospital out-patient departments more heavily than Whites do. One is related to insurance status. The 20% of Blacks who lack health insurance probably seek medical care infrequently, especially if they also are among the one third of Black Americans who are poor. Infrequent use of medical services is related to lack of a regular physician, and people who lack a regular provider to advise them in the course of treatment often seek services inappropriately—for example, going to an emergency room with a head cold. Another reason Blacks may frequent hospital outpatient departments is their hours of operation. Making and keeping appointments within a 9 to 5 workday is hard for people who work the graveyard shift or shifts with irregular hours. Lower-income people are more likely to work such shifts. Despite legendarily long waits in some emergency rooms, some feel the care in hospital outpatient departments is superior to the care received in the office of a solo practitioner, mainly because of the ready access to high-tech equipment and an array of specialists that this locale offers.

Disease and Mortality

Among both Whites and African Americans, life expectancy (or expected remaining years of life) from birth is greater for women than men. However, racial disparity overlays this as well, with the life expectancy for White females (nearly 80 years) exceeding that for Black females (74 years), and the life expectancies of both Black and White females exceeding those of Black males (65 years) and White males (73 years), respectively (NCHS, 1995).

This section reviews the facts about selected conditions that reduce the quality of life and often lessen life expectancy for African American women. Excess deaths reflect the number of deaths that would not have occurred if African Americans experienced the same age and sex death rates as Whites. According to the 1985 *Secretary's Report on*

Black and Minority Health, nearly 80% of the excess deaths among Blacks less than 70 years of age were caused by the following conditions: cardiovascular disease (41%); infant mortality (12%); cancer (10%); homicide (6%); diabetes (3%); cirrhosis of the liver (3%); and accidents (1%). In keeping with this finding, the disease conditions examined in this chapter for Black women include hypertension and heart disease, cancer, diabetes, unintentional injuries, and HIV/AIDS.

HYPERTENSION/HEART DISEASE/
CEREBROVASCULAR DISEASE

People are classified as hypertensive if their average systolic blood pressure is greater than 140 mm mercury, or their average diastolic blood pressure is greater than 90 mm mercury, or if they report taking high blood pressure medicine. Hypertension is a major risk factor for coronary heart disease and cerebrovascular disease, the major causes of death among women (and men) in the United States. It affects the health of Black women much more than it does the health of White women. Based on data collected from 1988 to 1991, 31% of Black women were found to be hypertensive, more than 1.6 times the rate among White females (19%) (NCHS, 1995).

Between 1950 and 1981, the death rate for Black women from heart disease decreased by 45%; the death rate from cerebrovascular disease decreased by 63% over the same period (Headen & Headen, 1985-1986). In spite of these trends, in 1985, the age- and sex-adjusted death rates from heart disease for Black women were 50% higher than for White women (Leffall, 1990). In 1992, the same pattern prevailed. Diseases of the heart caused 98 age-adjusted deaths per 100,000 White females that year, while causing 162 age-adjusted deaths per 100,000 Black females (NCHS, 1995) (see Table 8.1).

If we look at potential years of life lost per 100,000 population under 65 years of age, the toll taken on African American women by heart disease becomes even more apparent. In 1992, Black women lost 797 years of life to heart disease while White women lost 305 years of life (NCHS, 1995) (see Table 8.2).

Cerebrovascular diseases (including stroke) caused 23 deaths per 100,000 White females and 40 deaths per 100,000 Black females in 1992 (Table 8.1). The racial differential is magnified when potential

Table 8.1 Death Rates (per 100,000 Population) From Selected Causes for Females, by Race, 1992

Selected Causes	Black Females	White Females
Diseases of the heart	162.4	98.1
Cerebrovascular diseases	39.9	22.5
Cancers		
Respiratory system	28.5	27.4
Breast	27.0	21.7
Diabetes Mellitus	25.8	9.6
Unintentional injuries	19.3	16.1
Motor vehicle accidents	8.7	9.6
HIV/AIDS infection	14.3	1.6

SOURCE: NCHS, 1995.

Table 8.2 Years of Potential Life Lost Before Age 65 (per 100,000 Population) From Selected Causes of Death for Females, by Race, 1992

Selected Causes	Black Females	White Females
Diseases of the heart	796.7	305.4
Cerebrovascular diseases	220.4	79.9
Cancers		
Respiratory system	154.6	149.1
Breast	271.2	205.6
Diabetes mellitus	126.4	51.6
Unintentional injuries	590.1	438.0
Motor vehicle accidents	298.0	297.0
HIV/AIDS infection	462.3	51.7

SOURCE: NCHS, 1995.

years of life lost before age 65 are examined, however. Cerebrovascular disease caused the loss of 80 years of life per 100,000 White women less than 65 years of age in 1992. It was responsible for the loss of 220 years of life among Black women—2.75 times the years of potential life lost for White women (NCHS, 1995) (Table 8.2).

CANCER

Cancer is the second leading cause of death for women in the United States (second to heart disease), and, although White women have higher incidences of most types of cancers than Black women, Black women have higher death rates and lower 5-year survival rates than White women for most types of cancer (Horton, 1992). For example, the 5-year survival rate for White women with breast cancer is greater than 70%, but it is only 64% for Black women (Horton, 1992).

Since 1987, the major cause of cancer deaths among White women has been lung cancer (NCHS, 1991). In 1992, cancers of the respiratory system (including the lung) were responsible for 27 deaths per 100,000 White females, while breast cancer caused 22 deaths per 100,000. For Black women, in 1992, breast and respiratory system cancers caused nearly the same number of deaths: 28 African American women per 100,000 died of breast cancer and 29 died of respiratory system cancer (NCHS, 1995) (Table 8.1).

Although the same number of potential years of life (close to 150 per 100,000 population less than 65 years of age) were lost by Black and White women from respiratory system cancers, Black women less than 65 years of age lost a greater number of potential years of life (271 years) from breast cancer than did White women (206 years) (NCHS, 1995) (Table 8.2). This no doubt reflects the greater incidence of breast cancer among Black women at earlier ages and the lower survival rates for Black women who get cancer.

Cancer of the cervix and of the uterus also take a large toll on African American women, for whom the incidences remain twice as high as for White women (Horton, 1992). In addition, the 5-year relative survival rate for African American women (57%) from cervical cancer is 10 percentage points lower than the comparable rate for White women (67%) (Horton, 1992). For uterine cancer, the 5-year survival rate among Black women is 29 percentage points lower than that for White women—55% versus 84% (Horton, 1992).

DIABETES MELLITUS

Diabetes mellitus, a chronic condition characterized by abnormal glucose metabolism, is a major health problem for African American women. Diabetes primarily affects the circulatory system and is frequently associated with conditions such as arteriosclerosis (hardening of the arteries) and kidney failure. The incidence of diabetes among Black women is double that for White women—51 per 1,000

Black women versus 23 per 1,000 White women in 1987 (Horton, 1992). Diabetes is often associated with obesity, and the patterns of obesity among Black and White female diabetics support this finding. About 83% of diabetic Black women aged 20 to 74 but only 62% of White women in the same age range are obese (Leffall, 1990).

Manifestations of diabetes during pregnancy also are more problematic for African American women than for White women. Although gestational diabetes (diabetes occurring in a pregnant woman) is present in 1% to 3% of all pregnancies in the White and Black populations, perinatal mortality (infant mortality at birth) for pregnant Black women with diabetes is three times higher than for pregnant White women with diabetes (Headen & Headen, 1985-1986).

The age-adjusted death rate from diabetes per 100,000 Black women in 1992 was 26, more than 2.6 times the rate for White women (9.6 per 100,000 population) (NCHS, 1995) (Table 8.1). White women lost 52 years of potential life per 100,000 population to diabetes in 1992, while Black women lost over twice as many years of potential life—126 (NCHS, 1995) (Table 8.2).

UNINTENTIONAL INJURIES

Unintentional injuries, including motor vehicular and other accidents, are less significant causes of impairment and death among women than they are among men. These accidental injuries also cause fewer deaths than do hypertension and heart disease, cancer, and diabetes mellitus. In 1992, equal numbers of deaths per 100,000 Black and White women—that is, 19 and 16, respectively—were attributable to unintentional injuries. Nine of the 19 deaths per 100,000 Black women were specifically due to motor vehicle accidents, as were 10 of the 16 deaths per 100,000 among White women (NCHS, 1995) (Table 8.1).

These relatively small numbers of deaths per 100,000 women translate into sizable numbers of potential years of life lost per 100,000 Black and White women less than 65 years of age, primarily because accidental deaths are more common at younger ages. Among Black women less than 65 years of age, 590 potential years of life were lost per 100,000 women, whereas 438 years were lost by White women (NCHS, 1995) (Table 8.2).

HIV/AIDS

Although the reported patterns of transmission of the human immunodeficiency virus (HIV) that causes acquired immune deficiency syndrome (AIDS) vary by racial and ethnic group, all women have been affected by this disease. The number of cases reported among African American women age 13 and over for all the years data have been collected was 21,707, whereas 10,288 cases were reported among White women (NCHS, 1994). As these figures suggest, Black women are overrepresented in the proportion of reported HIV/AIDS cases when compared to their proportion in the total female population, and White women are underrepresented. Although Black women account for only 13.3% of all women, they account for nearly three fifths of all HIV/AIDS cases among women. White women account for 75% of all women ages 15 to 44 but report only 25% of the HIV/AIDS cases. According to Selik, Castro, and Pappaioanou (1988), AIDS is 13.2 times more common among Black women than among White women.

When female AIDS cases reported through October 1991 were examined by method of transmission, for both Black and White women, the dominant mode of infection was intravenous drug use—56% for Black women and 42% for White women. The second most common mode of transmission (heterosexual contact) was reported by nearly equal shares of Black and White women—34% and 31%, respectively—and blood transfusion (the third source of AIDS infection) showed greater disparity by race. Only 3% of Black women but 20% of White women reported this source (Asian American Health Forum, 1992).

The risk of transmission by sex between women seems to be lower than the risk of transmission via same-gender sex among men or via sex between men and women. Thus, data on transmission by sex between women are not reported separately, and lesbians may not engage in "safe sex" because of the protection they presume their "low-risk" status for HIV/AIDS affords them. Lesbians who are intravenous drug users, however, can be the source of HIV infection among women (Young, Weissman, & Cohen, 1992).

Because it is difficult to conduct controlled experiments on intravenous drug users, this group of HIV/AIDS patients is less likely to be included in experimental protocols. This means that Black women may be somewhat less likely to receive antiviral medications in the future than other groups of HIV/AIDS patients, whose ranks are less dominated by intravenous drug users (Friedman et al., 1989).

Although heterosexual transmission is the second most frequently reported mode of HIV/AIDS infection for both White and Black women, Black women may be more vulnerable than White women to heterosexual transmission of HIV/AIDS through sex with bisexual men. This may occur because, compared to White gay men, a larger proportion of Black gay men report having sex with both men and women—30% for Black and 13% for White gay men (Friedman et al., 1989).

When women have HIV/AIDS, others in their households—lovers, spouses, and/or children—also are likely to have the disease. Women with AIDS who must also fulfill their traditional roles as caregivers have shorter life expectancies than women who do not have the added stress of providing care to others. In addition, women with AIDS often leave behind orphans with HIV/AIDS, many of whom subsequently are raised by their grandmothers, a fact that increases the stresses in the lives of these older women. The age-adjusted death rate in 1992 per 100,000 Black women from HIV/AIDS is 14, compared to the death rate of 2 per 100,000 White women (NCHS, 1995) (Table 8.1).

Health Reform to Improve
the Health of African American Women

So far this chapter has reported on many factors that influence the health outcomes of African American women. As the Congress and the President seek to reform the national health care delivery system—just one variable in the "health equation" for us all—they should be mindful of the components of access to health care services and should strive to make access meaningful for all.

Access to health care services is defined as having health insurance coverage (either employer-based or government-funded) and, thereby, being able to get user-friendly medical care delivered by a culturally competent provider in a conveniently located facility whenever needed and at an affordable price. The lack of insurance coverage and dependence on insurance coverage such as Medicaid, which may not guarantee the ability to get user-friendly medical care, have been noted above as impediments to access to care. Thus, reform proposals should aim to cover as many people as is affordable for the nation and to provide them genuine entrée to services.

The availability of culturally competent providers also is crucial to whether African American women actually seek care and follow through with the instructions given in a way that improves their health. Culturally competent providers are perceived by the members of a given culture as being knowledgeable and respectful of their mores, language, and styles of help seeking; they are, therefore, also perceived as valuable people from whom to seek health services. Although African American women, other women, and other African Americans, might be most likely to be perceived as culturally competent providers by African American women, the pool of appropriate providers must be made larger than that. Even with increasing numbers both of women and African Americans entering U.S. medical schools—currently 7.4% of students in U.S. medical schools are African Americans and about 40% are women—the day may never come when all African American women can have another African American woman as a physician for whatever her needs may be. Thus, into the indefinite future, to produce more culturally competent physicians, the need remains to incorporate awareness of health issues/needs of various subpopulations, such as African American women, into the training offered in U.S. medical schools. Health reform proposals would be wise to mandate this.

Location of medical facilities as a barrier to care also was noted in this chapter. Given the access problems both in urban and rural areas, the concept of placing all types of medical services, local social services agencies, and local offices of federal agencies (such as Social Security) at a single site warrants serious consideration. One-stop shopping for medical and other services would limit the transportation costs of getting care and might thereby increase the frequency of visits, ultimately improving health outcomes.

Both the issues of "whenever needed" and "at an affordable price" revolve around income. To address them, the reformed health care delivery system that evolves in this country should make it possible for all people to have access to appropriate care 24 hours per day and at a cost that is not going to cause the poorest of the poor to forgo needed treatment.

Conclusions

The burdens of racism, poverty, and lack of education, employment, and health insurance contribute to the morbidity and mortality of African American women, as do health habits and lifestyle. Conditions such as hypertension, heart disease, and cancer take their toll on these women, as do newer diseases such as HIV/AIDS.

Because the factors influencing the health of African American women are many, steps to improve the health of this subpopulation need to be taken in many arenas. Education (about health and for jobs) and employment are as necessary as medical care to reduce racial disparities in health for African American women. Policymakers need to keep this in mind as our nation considers reforming its system to finance and deliver health care.

References

Association of Asian Pacific Community Health Organizations. (n.d.). *Selected health and population statistics for Asians and Pacific Islanders.* Oakland: Author.

Calle, E. E., Flanders, D., Thun, M. J., & Martin, L. M. (1993). Demographic predictors of mammography and Pap smear screening in U.S. women. *American Journal of Public Health, 83,* 53-60.

Centers for Disease Control and Prevention. (1994). *HIV/AIDS Surveillance Report, 6*(2).

Communications Consortium Media Center & the National Council of Negro Women (n.d.). *The 1991-1992 women of color reproductive health poll.* Washington, DC: Authors.

Delgado, J. L., & Treviño, F. M. (1985). The state of Hispanic health in the United States. In *The state of Hispanic America* (Vol. 2, pp. 35-47). Oakland: National Hispanic Center for Advanced Studies and Policy Analysis.

Ewbank, D. C. (1989). History of Black mortality and health before 1940. In D. P. Willis (Ed.), *Health policies and Black Americans* (pp. 100-128). New Brunswick, NJ: Transaction.

Friedman, S. J., Sotheran, J. L., Abdul-Quader, A., Primm, B. J., Des Jarlais, D. C., Kleinman, P., Mauge, C., Goldsmith, D. S., El-Sadr, W., & Maslansky, R. (1989). The AIDS epidemic among Blacks and Hispanics. In D. P. Willis (Ed.), *Health policies and Black Americans* (pp. 455-499). New Brunswick, NJ: Transaction.

Headen, A. E., Jr., & Headen, S. W. (1985-1986). General health conditions and medical insurance issues concerning Black women. *Review of Black Political Economy, 14,* 183-197.

Hogue, C. J. R., & Hargraves, M. A. (1993). Class, race, and infant mortality in the United States. *American Journal of Public Health, 83,* 9-12.

Horton, J. A. (Ed.). (1992). *The women's health data book: A profile of women's health in the United States.* Washington, DC: Jacobs Institute of Women's Health.

Jaynes, G. D., & Williams, R. M. (1989). Black Americans' health. In G. D. Jaynes & R. M. Williams (Eds.), *A common destiny: Blacks and American society* (pp. 391-450). Washington, DC: National Academy Press.

Leffall, L. D. (1990). Health status of Black Americans. In *The state of Black America 1990* (pp. 121-142). New York: National Urban League.

Leigh, W. A. (1994a). The health status of women of color. In C. Costello & A. J. Stone (Eds.), *The American woman 1994-95: Women and health* (pp. 154-196). New York: Norton.

Leigh, W. A. (1994b). *Housing and neighborhood characteristics by race and ethnicity.* Washington, DC: Joint Center for Political and Economic Studies for the Ford Foundation.

Liu, W. T., & Yu, E. S. H. (1985). Ethnicity, mental health, and the urban delivery system. In L. Maldonado & J. Moore (Eds.), *Urban ethnicity in the United States* (pp. 211-247). Beverly Hills, CA: Sage.

Manton, K. G., Patrick, C. H., & Johnson, K. W. (1989). Health differentials between Blacks and Whites: Recent trends in mortality and morbidity. In D. P. Willis (Ed.), *Health policies and Black Americans* (pp. 129-189). New Brunswick, NJ: Transaction.

Miller, S. M. (1989). Race in the health of America. In D. P. Willis (Ed.), *Health policies and Black Americans* (pp. 500-531). New Brunswick, NJ: Transaction.

National Center for Health Statistics (NCHS). (1991). *Health, United States, 1990.* Hyattsville, MD: Public Health Service.

National Center for Health Statistics (NCHS). (1995). *Health, United States, 1994.* Hyattsville, MD: Public Health Service.

National Council of La Raza. (1992). *Hispanics and health insurance: Vol.2. Analysis and policy implications.* Washington, DC: Labor Council for Latin American Advancement and National Council of La Raza.

National Institute on Drug Abuse. (1994). *Summary tables: Annualized estimates from the national pregnancy and health survey.* Rockville, MD: Author.

Rice, M. F., & Winn, M. (1991). Black health care and the American health system: A political perspective. In T. J. Litman & L. S. Robins (Eds.), *Health politics and policy* (pp. 320-334). New York: Delmar.

Schoendorf, K. C., Hogue, C. J. R., Kleinman, J. C., & Rowley, D. (1992). Mortality among infants of Black as compared with White college-educated parents. *New England Journal of Medicine, 326,* 1522-1526.

Selik, R. M., Castro, K. G., & Pappaioanou, M. (1988). Racial/ethnic differences in the risk of AIDS in the United States. *American Journal of Public Health, 78,* 1539-1544.

Short, P. F., Cornelius, L. J., & Goldstone, D. E. (1990). Health insurance of minorities in the United States. *Journal of Health Care for the Poor and Underserved, 1,* 9-24.

Smith, G. D., & Egger, M. (1992). Socioeconomic differences in mortality in Britain and the United States. *American Journal of Public Health, 82,* 1079-1081.

Stevens, J., Kumanyika, S. K., & Keil, J. E. (1994). Attitudes toward body size and dieting: Differences between elderly Black and White women. *American Journal of Public Health, 84,* 1322-1325.

U.S. Bureau of the Census. (1992a). *The Black population in the United States: March 1991* (Current population reports, Series P-20, No. 464). Washington, DC: Government Printing Office.

U.S. Bureau of the Census. (1992b). *Health insurance: Who was covered between 1987 and 1990?* (Statistical Brief SB/92-8). Washington, DC: U.S. Department of Commerce.

U.S. Bureau of the Census. (1992c). *Statistical abstract of the United States: 1992* (112th ed.). Washington, DC: Government Printing Office.

U.S. Bureau of the Census. (1993). *Statistical abstract of the United States: 1993* (113th ed.). Washington, DC: Government Printing Office.

U.S. Department of Health and Human Services. (1985). *Report of the secretary's task force on Black and minority health.* Washington, DC: Author.

U.S. Department of Health and Human Services. (n.d.). *Wellness for women: Issues in women's health care today.* Washington, DC: Author.

Wilkinson, D. Y., & King, G. (1989). Conceptual and methodological issues in the use of race as a variable: Policy implications. In D. P. Willis (Ed.), *Health policies and Black Americans* (pp. 56-71). New Brunswick, NJ: Transaction.

Young, R. M., Weissman, G., & Cohen, J. B. (1992). Assessing risk in the absence of information: HIV risk among women injection-drug users who have sex with women. *AIDS & Public Policy Journal, 7,* 175-183.

9 Arab Middle Eastern American Women
Stereotyped, Invisible, but Powerful

AFAF IBRAHIM MELEIS

MARIANNE HATTAR-POLLARA

M iddle Eastern is a term often used to identify people who originated in the Middle East region of the world. Although a large
majority of countries in the Middle East are Arab countries, not all
Middle Eastern Americans are Arabs. Some come from non-Arab Middle Eastern countries, such as Turkey, Iran, Afghanistan, and Pakistan,
and are considered Middle Eastern Americans. Other ethnic minorities, such as Armenians, Assyrians, and Chaldenians, who once lived
in the Arab Middle East, maintained their own ethnic identity rather
than a regional identity, and they are referred to by ethnicity most of
the time (Lipson, Reizian, & Meleis, 1987).

Political changes over the course of the century have shaped,
defined, and redefined the identity of Arab Middle Eastern immigrants in the United States. Prior to World War I, the Arab Middle
East was ruled by the Ottoman Empire; thus the early waves of
immigrants who arrived from the Ottoman province of Greater Syria
(now divided into Jordan, Syria, Lebanon, and Palestine) tended to

133

identify themselves as Syrians (Haddad, 1983; Naff, 1983). As the Arab countries gained independence, "incoming immigrants identified themselves according to the nation-state from which they originated" (Abraham, 1983, p. 98). Changes in identity among immigrants from this part of the world also occurred after the 1948 Israeli-Arab war. A pan-Arab nationalist movement emerged during the Nasserite era (1953-1970), leading immigrants to identify themselves as Arabs first, before their identification with a country of origin (Wigle & Abraham, 1974). With subsequent political upheavals and following the defeat of the Arab states in the 1967 Arab-Israeli war, pan-Arab nationalistic sentiment vanished and was replaced by a country-of-origin identity (Abraham, 1983). During the last decade, Arab-American identity seemed to be the one that made immigrants from the Arab Middle East and their offspring most comfortable. This ethnic identity "allows its members to emphasize the common features of their Arab history, culture, and language, on the one side, and the common themes which bind them in their American experience on the other" (Abraham, 1983, p. 100).

In this chapter, the term *Middle Eastern immigrant women in the United States* refers to women who immigrated from any of the Arab countries in the Middle East, as well as female descendants of Arab Middle Eastern immigrants who identify themselves as either Arab Americans, Arab Middle Eastern Americans, or natives of a specific Arab Middle Eastern country (e.g., Lebanese American, Jordanian American). The Arab Middle East extends from the Arabian Gulf in Asia to the Atlantic coast in Africa, an area half as large as that of the United States. Arab Middle Eastern American women may have originated from any of the following Arab countries. According to Omran (1980),

Morocco, Mauritania, Algeria, Tunisia, and Libya, which are located in North Africa;

Egypt, the Sudan, and Somalia, which are located in the Nile Valley and the African Horn;

Syria, Lebanon, Jordan, Iraq, and Palestine, which are located in the Fertile Crescent; and

Saudi Arabia, the two Yemens, Oman, the United Arab Emirates, Qatar, Bahrain, and Kuwait, which are located in the Arab Peninsula and Gulf Region.

For over a century, sizable and growing immigration to the United States has occurred from the Arab Middle East (Naff, 1983). In spite of their history and their large numbers in the United States, there is a dearth of health-related knowledge about them in general and about Arab Middle Eastern American women in particular. Systematic studies that would provide important information about their demographic distribution, their health behavior, and their health risks and needs, as well as related morbidity and mortality data, are nonexistent. This chapter will focus on providing a context to help health care professionals to understand the health concerns and health needs of Arab Middle Eastern immigrant women in the United States. The specific purposes are to provide historical background for immigration of this group, describe their demographic profile, outline broadly some of the structural and cultural stressors that women confront, describe their health and illness experiences and relevant coping strategies, and define the issues they encounter in using health care resources.

Immigration History

Although selective immigration of Arab Middle Eastern individuals dates back as far as the 15th century (Mehdi, 1978), it was not until the 1880s and 1900s that Arab Middle Easterners began immigrating in significant numbers. Between 1880 and 1938, an estimated 250,000 Arabs entered the United States (Nigem, 1986). Immigration occurred in phases and waves and was heavily influenced by the economic and political situation at areas of origin and in the United States (Haddad, 1983; Nigem, 1986). Their pattern of immigration, their demographic composition, and the motivating factors for immigration can be divided into two major time periods, each including several waves of immigration. The first (1876 to 1938) is referred to as the early immigration period. During this period, the overwhelming majority of Arab Middle Eastern immigrants to the United States came from what was called Greater Syria (Haddad, 1983). Arab Christian tradesmen, encouraged by the Ottoman sultan, came to exhibit Syrian wares at the Philadelphia International Exposition in 1876 (Naff, 1983). The combined impact of their enthusiastic reports, the recruiting activities of steamship agents for American industry, and the efforts of native brokers and money lenders led to a chain immigration from the Mount Lebanon area (Naff, 1983). The immigrants of this era were mostly uneducated, unskilled peasants of low socioeconomic status (Haddad, 1983).

In the late 19th century, the Ottoman Empire was replaced by a Turkish revolutionary government. When this new government made military service mandatory for Christians as well as Moslems, significantly more Christian Arabs immigrated to the United States to escape military service (Naff, 1983). Initially, Moslem Arabs were less likely to immigrate to the United States for fear that they would be unable to maintain their Islamic traditions in a Western Christian society (Haddad, 1983; Naff, 1983), "but continuing success stories of other immigrants provided the necessary incentive" (Haddad, 1983, p. 66). By 1918 to 1922, significant numbers of young, single Arab Moslem men were entering the United States to work in the Ford Rouge plant in Dearborn, Michigan (Wasfi, 1971). These bachelors were soon followed by married men and families. Most were small tradesmen, artisans, and skilled laborers; only a handful were intellectuals or professionals.

Thus, although most of the first wave of immigrants during the early period were young single males, later waves included women and families. Between 1899 and 1915, about 47% of Arab immigrants in the United States were women, and in the 1920s, women immigrants outnumbered men (Naff, 1983). The restrictive Immigration Act of 1924, the Great Depression, and World War II severely curbed immigration between 1925 and 1947 (Abraham, 1983; Haddad, 1983). A large percentage of these early immigrants settled in southern states, about 25% remained in the East, and about the same percentage moved to the Midwest (Elkholy, 1969; Younis, 1961). These immigrants were Palestinians, Iraqis, Egyptians, Yemenites, and Moroccans, along with the immigrants from Greater Syria.

The second period of immigration, beginning around 1947, was characterized by political events such as the Palestinian problem, which resulted from the creation of the State of Israel, and the subsequent wars that followed, including the Lebanese crisis. All of these political events contributed to the second wave of immigration (Nigem, 1986), which significantly increased the number of Arab Americans in the United States, particularly those who were Moslems and who left Palestine after the Israeli Palestinian war.

The liberalization of immigration laws in 1965, which took effect in 1968, allowed Arab immigrants from many Middle Eastern countries to arrive in large numbers (Abraham, 1983). This period is characterized by a third wave of immigrants. These immigrants were largely professionals with strong educational backgrounds (Nigem, 1986), part of a "brain drain" that reached its peak between 1968 and 1971 (Abraham, 1983; Nigem, 1986). Census data estimate that 154,000 Arab immigrants arrived between 1949 and 1976 (Naff, 1980). The post-1968 wave of immigrants included a higher proportion of Moslems, females, married, educated, and skilled people than previous waves. These immigrants tended to settle in large urban areas (Elkholy, 1969; Mehdi, 1978; Naff, 1980; Younis, 1961).

Demographic Profile

Significant discrepancies exist between official and unofficial estimates of the Arab Middle Eastern immigrant population in the United States, depending on the source of the estimate. Informal and unofficial estimates by Arab American organizations and Arab American scholars indicate a population of 1 to 3 million (Mehdi, 1978; Naff, 1980). The U.S. Bureau of the Census (1979) estimated 480,000 (U.S. Bureau of the Census, 1979), while the 1980 Census estimate was 660,000. The 1990 Census data count 716,391 first-generation Arab Middle Eastern Americans and 154,347 of the second-generation (U.S. Bureau of the Census, 1990). Immigration and Naturalization Service records indicate that 367,160 immigrants from Iraq, Jordan, Lebanon, Egypt, and Syria were naturalized between 1961 and 1990 (U.S. Bureau of the Census, 1990). Such large discrepancies, according to Nigem (1986), are due to sampling and nonsampling errors. The sampling error of the 1979 *Current Population Survey* was large, especially when estimating small sample-size populations. Nonsampling errors also have resulted in lower estimates, and these were mainly due to the bureau's focus on large groups. Evidence of methodological problems was also observed in the difference of about 180,000 between the 1979 and 1980 census estimates (Nigem, 1986).

Discrepancies are attributed to conceptual and pragmatic issues. The U.S. Bureau of the Census's Statistical Policy Directive No. 15, issued by the U.S. Office of Management and Budget, does not recognize Arab Middle Eastern Americans as a separate category. Immigrants from the Arab Middle East are grouped together under the "others" category (U.S. Bureau of the Census, 1992). Therefore, demographic health-related data are nonexistent. Nigem (1986) conducted an analysis of Arab Middle Eastern immigrants in the United States, using the 1979 *Current Population Survey* and the 1980 Census Bureau data. His analysis revealed that a large portion of Arab Middle Eastern Americans are foreign born (53.7%). Of the foreign born, a large portion (54%) entered the United States recently (1970 to 1979), and about 45% are naturalized. About 54.3% of Arab Middle Easterners spoke a language other than English at home. About 86% spoke English well, compared to 80% of the overall U.S. population. The distribution by region showed that 30.4% resided in the Northeast, 27.2% in the North Central states, 21.6% in the South, and the remaining 20.8% in the West. A large percentage of Arab Middle Eastern immigrants lived in metropolitan areas, about 81.5%, compared to 69.3% of the total U.S. population. Of these, 36.6% lived in central cities, compared to 19.5% of the U.S. population (Nigem, 1986).

Nigem's (1986) analysis also revealed that over 50% of Arab Middle Eastern immigrants in the United States have some higher education, compared to 34% of the U.S. population. The high rates of higher education (college and graduate work) were explained partially in terms of the large proportion of foreign born. Of the foreign-born Arab Middle Easterners, 27.7% completed 4 years or more of college education, compared to 15.8% of all foreign-born Americans, and 16.2% of the total U.S. population. About 61% of Arab Middle Eastern immigrants in the United States have white-collar occupations, compared to 49.4% of the U.S. population; they also have a high rate of professionals (20%).

The median income for Arab Middle Easterners in the United States is $19,950, compared to $15,800 for the U.S. population. Also, 29.5% earn more than $25,000, compared to 23.3% of the U.S. population. With respect to other demographic variables, such as age, sex, and marital status, Nigem (1986) indicated that little difference existed with respect to age between this population and the U.S.

population. Slightly higher proportions of the overall U.S. population were age 65 or older and under the age of 14, (10.9% and 22.4%,
compared to 8.0% and 19.9% of Arab Middle Easterners). A high
male-to-female ratio was observed for Arab Middle Easterners in the
United States (105), compared to the U.S. population (91.9), indicating that more males than females have immigrated to the United
States from the Arab Middle East. Also due to selective immigration,
Arab Middle Easterners had a lower proportion of people who had
never married than the U.S. population.

Arab Middle Eastern immigrant women in the United States constitute a unique and a distinct ethnic group, sharing common social,
cultural, linguistic, and demographic traits, a similar outlook on life,
and similar aspirations. They come from countries that are strikingly
similar in terms of high rate of population growth, a young population structure, a high rate of marriage, an early age at marriage, a
large family size norm, and an agrarian, rural-oriented community
life. They also experienced and were exposed to similar health patterns in their countries of origin, where communicable diseases lead
the causes of morbidity and mortality. Childhood and maternal
mortality rates are generally high, and life expectancy is moderate in
most of the Arab countries (Omran, 1980).

Despite these common characteristics that define their ethnic identity, these women tend to vary in other characteristics, such as
religion, sociopolitical background, and immigration experience. In
the Arab Middle East, about 90% of the population are either Sunni
or Shi'ite Moslems. The remaining 10% are Christians, either Roman
Catholic, Greek Orthodox, or Protestant. The percentages are almost
exactly reversed among those Arab Middle Easterners who have
immigrated to the United States; about 90% are Christians of different orientations, and the remaining 10% are Moslems (Naff, 1983).
No data are readily available to update these ratios. Both Moslems
and Christians, however, share similar ethnic aspirations and community living (Omran, 1980).

Arab Middle Eastern immigrant women come from 20 independent Arab countries, as well as from Palestine; these countries vary
extensively in wealth and in sociopolitical history with regard to the
women's movement and women's education and participation in the
labor force. Thus, Arab Middle Eastern immigrant women present a

diverse picture in terms of socioeconomic status, level of education, occupation, and level of acculturation and assimilation. Some have come with established wealth, whereas others still struggle to realize the American dream. Some are professionals and career-oriented; others are less educated and may be unemployed; some may subscribe only to traditional values, and others may adopt Western values.

The factors that motivated their immigration to the United States also vary. Although the majority came to join other family members in chain immigration, some came seeking higher education and remained, others came seeking a better quality of life for themselves and their children, and still others were either displaced by war as refugees or immigrated to escape a war situation or an oppressive regime (Lipson & Meleis, 1983; Meleis, 1981). Given all of these factors, and in the absence of systematic research studies, it can only be assumed that the health responses and health needs of these women will vary accordingly.

The participation of Arab American women in the U.S. workforce is substantial but not well-documented. For example, most Palestinian, Jordanian, Lebanese, and Syrian women help their spouses manage family-owned or family-run businesses. However, such work is rarely reported by women as employment, unless it is for tax reasons. Furthermore, because of language barriers, some Arab American women conduct their business at home. This is usually in the form of handmade crafts, which include sewing, needlepoint, and the like. Working in a family business is considered an extension of the women's duties as a wife and as a mother. Fouad (1986) indicated that most employed Middle Eastern immigrant women are working in family businesses. The impact of such employment, or the extension of duties as wife and mother, on the family dynamics is not known, and this area needs to be studied.

Immigration and Stress

Overall, Arab Middle Eastern immigrant women view their settlement in the United States favorably, despite the many losses they incurred in terms of social status, family network and ties, and social support, as well as the difficulties they encounter in terms of cultural, linguistic, and social barriers (Hattar-Pollara & Meleis, in press). They value the numerous resources that facilitate their daily functions, the many opportunities for growth, the educational opportunities for their children, and the quality of life that challenges them and their families to move forward. Nonetheless, Arab Middle Eastern women have been shaped by a unique cultural, historical, and religious tradition. Within this tradition, they have developed their own cultural values, their own definition of role functions and role responsibilities, and their own definition of power and status—all of these are very different from those held by women in the West. As immigrant women they experience increasing role overload and stress related to new demands occasioned by their efforts to meeting competing sets of expectations in the new host country (Hattar-Pollara & Meleis, 1995). Arab Middle Eastern immigrant women, by virtue of being immigrants and women from Arab Middle Eastern countries that value conformity, tend to suffer from stressors situated within the family and stressors germane to their immigrant status in a Western society. They experience structural and cultural stressors.

STRUCTURAL STRESSORS

Stereotyping. Recent studies have demonstrated that Arab Middle Eastern immigrant women tend to suffer from stereotypes, stigma, misunderstanding, and social isolation (Hattar-Pollara & Meleis, 1995; Meleis, 1991), all of which have serious consequences on their health, on their health risk, and their health needs. The media have not been kind to Middle Eastern immigrants, to Arabs, or to women. When all three attributes are combined, as in Arab Middle Eastern immigrants, the outcome is more serious. Mention an Arab woman to a health care professional and the immediate image is of a subservient, powerless, and abused voiceless creature. When these health care professionals are confronted by a seemingly articulate, outspoken, and forceful woman, their reactions range from shock to another form of stereotyping.

Health care providers tend to give more attention to those clients who demonstrate outward symbols of Americanization. Less assertive Arab women feel that they are ignored, devalued, and provided with less than adequate health care. Although Americanization might be seen by the American culture as the ultimate goal for every immigrant, being and becoming Americanized is avoided by Middle Eastern women. Becoming Americanized means being ostracized by their community and alienated from their social network. Being Americanized means that they have traded their own cultural values for those their culture believes represent societal and familial disintegration. Middle Eastern immigrants see being Americanized—*Itamrak*—as becoming individualistic, or selfish, and putting oneself over others. It means valuing time and punctuality over people's needs. It means becoming an aggressive woman, and it means that a woman has become disloyal to her own people. A person who is Itamrak is viewed with mixed emotions. On the one hand, she is admired for being able to move on, but on the other, she is condemned for appearing to have sold her soul to become "one of them" rather than "one of us." Americanization of immigrants denotes a loss of identity. Some Middle Eastern women's dilemmas can be understood within this concept of Americanization. The American identity is feared and avoided. Biculturalism is what they strive for.

If stereotyping is replaced by the concept of diversity, then the uniqueness of the individual emerges in the health care encounter and individualization of care can occur. In spite of what they may be wearing or how they respond, Arab women in the United States are businesswomen, professionals, and proactive homemakers. They are physicians, lawyers, nurses, entrepreneurs, politicians, farm workers, and small-business workers. If they appear modest, then their modesty represents their cultural upbringing and perhaps their religious teaching. This modesty can be mistaken for powerlessness and gender-based oppression. Although this may be true in some situations, another oppression described by Arab Middle Easterners is oppression of stereotyping. Understanding their context requires accepting their biculturalism, their diversity, as well as their similarities.

Politicism. A second structural stressor shares the same properties of prejudice, discrimination, and racism (Meleis, Dallafar, & Lipson, 1995). One of the most revealing findings, in a study of medical records for Arab American patients, was the inaccurate recording of their national and cultural heritage by health care professionals

(Lipson, Reizian, & Meleis, 1987). In their conclusions, the authors expressed concern about health care professionals who may have demonstrated their "geographical ignorance" and "cultural insensitivity" by confusing Arabs, Latin Americans, Africans, and Middle Easterners. Since this study was completed, extensive clinical work with Arab Middle Eastern immigrants has led to a different interpretation of this erroneous and misguided information. The term *politicism* refers to bias based on politics and religion that leads to acts such as recording misinformation like that described above. (Meleis, 1993). Politicism shares some of the properties of racism, but the origins are different. Racism is discrimination and stigmatization rooted in race and color of skin; politicism is based on politics and religion. Arab women are reluctant to identify their country of origin because of Middle Eastern politics. They evade or ignore the question of their country of origin, or they may misinform interviewers. They fear that if they share the truth, they will be subjected to discrimination, denial of service, and/or humiliation. They attribute this to politics and religion. The results of politicism are similar to racism. Politicism makes them reluctant to keep appointments, to follow a health regimen, to ask questions, or to comply.

CULTURAL STRESSORS

Not all stressors in the life of immigrant Arab women are attributed to structural constraints in the new society. The values, norms, expectations, and sanctions of their native culture create another set of stressors. The most pertinent cultural stressors are familialism and rumors.

Familialism. Middle Eastern women share a commitment to family orientation. Whether this orientation is due to a lengthy socialization process or is coerced can be debated. The net result is that to understand Arab women's triumphs and tribulations, one has to come to grips with what it means for an Arab woman to have a family of origin, a family of in-laws, and a family of one's own. When European Americans speak of a family, they usually refer to the nuclear family; when a Middle Eastern woman refers to a family, it usually includes her parents, siblings, aunts and uncles, cousins, in-laws, and those friends who have become like family. Families give support when needed, but they also deliver sanctions with the same zeal. Families are supposed to keep individuals in line, to prevent them from losing their own cultural values and becoming Americanized. Familialism is a buffer against stress, but it is also a cause of stress. Families congregate together to support a person who becomes ill—lack of family during illness episodes is a cause of distress. Because of the need for family support, immigrant women migrate back to their countries of origin. Familialism is a shield that prevents patients from learning the truth about their illness, and it prevents women from allowing the full integration of their children into the United States, because full integration means to them a loss of important values. When familialism is strong, Arab women are also prevented from forming new bonds with other communities. Because of familialism, medication courses are altered, diets are not followed, and health care practices are modified. To understand patterns of compliance with health promotion behaviors, we have to acknowledge the importance of familialism in the life of Arab women.

Middle Eastern women who migrate to the United States lose the support of their extended family and consequently may change or modify their roles (Meleis, Dallafar, & Lipson, 1995). Seeking employment is a case in point. Middle Eastern women who may never have worked before may find themselves in a position where taking a paid job is a matter of survival, or at least a matter of improving the family's living conditions. In such a case, instead of relying on family members to look after their children when they work—as they would in their country of origin—they have to seek outside help or redefine roles.

Among Middle Easterners, being a wife and a mother takes priority over being an employee. In this regard, employment does not provide women with a status that challenges or subordinates their roles as wives and mothers. To the contrary, in many cases, work may enforce these roles, by allowing women to redefine these roles in a more satisfying manner than existed prior to employment and U.S. residence (Pessar, 1984). A recent study on Jordanian immigrant women with adolescent children revealed that these women experienced constant pressure in managing their roles as wives, mothers, and members of their ethnic community. In their efforts to meet numerous new demands, and in their attempts to balance conflicting and competing sets of cultural and social expectations, they developed some creative approaches, managing their maternal role in a way that meets cultural expectations yet furthers the developmental needs of their adolescents and families (Hattar-Pollara & Meleis, 1995). In another study, conducted to describe the Arab American immigrant parents' social network and help-seeking behavior, May (1992) reported that although the extended family was perceived as the major source of support, parents thought they had smaller networks here and less support available from those networks than they had had in their home country. Loss of support was attributed to the long geographic distances from extended families and familiar network members.

Rumors: Community Talks (Kalam El Naas). In spite of the limited networks in the host country, there is a strong community hold. Rumors keep families in line, but rumors often prevent families from developing biculturalism to its fullest. Women are expected to promote and/or maintain the value systems they brought with them. Three concepts help women in that role:

1. *Adab,* that is, politeness and good behavior
2. *Eaib,* avoiding unacceptable behaviors
3. *Haram,* which differentiates between forbidden actions and sanctioned actions

Women are expected to carry on the tradition of vertical communication: The young respect and defer to adults, women respect and defer to men. Men, in return, are expected to protect women as fathers, brothers, male cousins, and sons. Immigrant women interface with U.S. systems more readily and tend to accept more horizontal and equal lines of authority. But their understanding of the significance of community expectations makes them vulnerable to conflicting demands.

Health and Illness

There are limited research data and findings related to the health and illness of Arab Middle Eastern immigrants in general and of women in particular. In the absence of more systematic approaches to determining their health and illness responses and factors that impinge on their health care, knowledge of their experiences in home countries, as well as clinical knowledge, will be used in this section. These findings should be used as a broad framework to understand their lived experiences in the United States rather than as specific guidelines for categorizing these experiences.

As stated earlier, this population is not accorded a separate category by the U.S. Bureau of the Census. Therefore, general or specific vital statistics about this population are nonexistent. Population studies conducted in the Arab Middle East can provide a context for understanding the situation of immigrants from that region. Omran (1980) surveyed and analyzed data pertaining to population growth, social and economic characteristics, fertility, morbidity and mortality, urbanization, and health in Arab Middle Eastern countries. The findings of his report will be used to illustrate relevant health patterns of immigrants.

Cross tabulation by age and sex indicated, with almost no exception, that Arab Middle Easterners who live in their country of origin are young in age. Taken as a whole, about 45% are under age 15, compared to 36% of the world population and only 25% of the population in the more developed countries. The percentage of the Arab population under 15 is even greater than that in the less developed countries, which is estimated to be 40%.

The older segment of the Arab population (those 65 years and older) is relatively small, constituting only 3% of the total, compared to 5.7% of the world population and 10.5% of the total in the more developed countries. The median age in Arab countries is about 17, compared to 22.4 worldwide and 30.2 in the more developed countries (Omran, 1980, p. 60).

With respect to sex, the ratio of males to females for all ages in the Arab populations is high, ranging from 103 to 105. This excess male composition, according to Omran (1980, p. 64), is either due to underreporting or to higher female mortality. Inaccurate reporting of the age of females contributes to distorting the sex ratio in certain age groups, for example, the age group 10 to 14. Females between the ages of 10 to 14 are often reported as being 15 to 20. There is also overreporting of females in other older age groups, which lowers the sex ratio in these groups.

The major health problems that characterize the less developed countries of the Arab Middle East and may influence immigrants' health are in mainly four areas: acute infectious diseases; parasitic diseases; certain deficiency diseases, such as iron deficiency and anemia of pregnancy, deficiency of iodine in water supplies, and protein-calorie malnutrition; and high infant, child, and maternal mortality rates.

With advancing health care systems in most of the Arab Middle East, new health problems have emerged. There is now an increasing prevalence of heart disease, hypertension, cerebrovascular diseases, cancer, diabetes, renal disease, and geriatric health problems (Omran, 1980, pp. 112-115). Data are not available to ascertain whether Arab Middle Eastern immigrants in the United States present similar patterns of health problems.

Health Beliefs and Practices

Hot and Cold. The Middle Eastern health belief system is based on the Hippocratic Galenic-Islamic tradition. The Arabs translated medical Greek texts, particularly those by Hippocrates and Galen, into Arabic, either directly or through Syriac. These texts were later translated from Arabic to Latin or other European languages, along with commentaries by the Arabs that helped correct many of Greek misconceptions and reinterpreted ambiguities in earlier explanations (Omran, 1980). The Islamic religion was also a stimulus to excel in medicine, as it made health a central concern, categorically rejecting magic and quackery and encouraging a search for a cure through the teachings of the Prophet, who declared: "Seek treatment, for there is no disease created by God for which He has not created a cure, except aging" (Omran, 1980, pp. 26-27).

On the basis of this tradition, the Arabs for a while adopted the Hippocratic theory of humoral pathology, according to which the physiology of human beings is determined by a balance between the four body humors and their qualities:

blood—hot and moist
yellow bile—hot and dry

phlegm—cold and moist
black bile—cold and dry

When all four humors are balanced, the body is healthy. When an imbalance occurs, an illness is manifested (Carrier, 1966). Also, each person has a unique temperament derived from a distinctive balance of the four humors. Temperament, which pertains here to the physical constitution rather than the personality, varies according to age (youth warmer, elderly colder), sex (females colder, males warmer), race, and climate (Pliskin, 1992). Arabs place more importance and emphasis on the "hot and cold" theory in practicing health maintenance and explaining illness causation. The main premise of the hot/cold theory is based on the notion that the healthy body is in a state of equilibrium in terms of the contrasting qualities of hot and cold. Exposure, either internally or externally, to excessive amounts of hot and cold is likely to cause disequilibrium. Traditionally, hot and cold are not determined simply by temperature, but by the qualities believed to be inherent in individuals and in particular substances such as food, herbs, medicine, and objects (Madsen, 1955, p. 23). Excessive ingestion of either cold or hot food can cause illness. It is not entirely clear nor consistently documented which types of food are cold and which are hot. However, upset stomach, distention, diarrhea, and constipation are ailments often attributed to system imbalance related to consumption of excessive amounts of either hot or cold food. Treatment remedies often entail preparing herbal hot drinks of either fresh mint leaves, boiled with water and sugar, or other herbs such as sage, chamomile, rosemary, and aniseed. Fresh mint boiled in water with sugar is believed to be an effective remedy for distention and constipation, and it is also often used with infants to treat colic pain. Chamomile and aniseed are believed to have similar effects, but they are also used for their calming effect on the nerves—often to help infants fall asleep. Sage is used mostly for stomach pain, stomach upset, and diarrhea. It is believed to restore the natural balance of the stomach and strengthen the inner mucosal lining of the intestine to stop diarrhea. Rosemary alone or with sage is also used for intestinal cramps and menstrual pain. Boiled cumin is used to relieve stomachs and intestines from distension and gas pain.

Winds, Drafts, and Currents. Arab Middle Easterners believe that drafts, winds, and currents expose the body to illness. The basis of this belief seems to be built upon the early Greco-Islamic tradition. Exposure to drafts can cause muscular stiffness and other aches and pains, such as pain in the joints or stomach upset, as well as nasal or intestinal colds. Drafts are particularly dangerous for menstruating and postpartum women because changing the body temperature by exposure to drafts may affect the normal flow of the menstrual blood. Moving from a warm place to a cold place, getting the body wet in the rain, and having wet shoes may cause a range of illnesses, including sneezing, runny nose, sore throat, chest cold and congestion, cough, and fever. It is believed that the body is particularly vulnerable to drafts and winds when the pores are open, while wounds are healing, or while a person is recuperating from surgery.

A similar belief system is found among Italian Americans. Ragucci (1981) indicates that Italian Americans guard and protect themselves and their dependents from exposure to atmospheric conditions, and they believe that a person who is perspiring is in a particularly dangerous state because the pores are more open. The term used in Arabic for these conditions is *lafhet hawa* or *akhadit bard* (struck by the wind), and on the basis of such belief, infants are usually covered with several layers of clothing before they are taken outside the house; postpartum women may refuse to be situated in a room where there is a draft; parents wrap their children's stomach areas before they go to bed, to avoid the possibility of their catching a stomach cold if the bed cover falls off; and, menstruating women are advised not to take baths while having their period. (The latter practice is now confined to the most rural areas.) Arab Middle Eastern women are reluctant sometimes to take baths during the first few postpartum days (Meleis & Sorell, 1981).

Some of the popular remedies for muscular stiffness, which is believed to be caused by drafts or sudden exposure to changes in atmospheric temperature, involve rubbing and massaging the afflicted area with hot oil or menthol-based ointment, or placing a menthol-based adhesive pad on the painful muscle. Drinking juices of citric fruits, especially hot lemonade, or drinking hot tea with honey is done to combat cold symptoms caused by exposure to changes in temperature. When cold symptoms become severe enough to cause persistent cough and chest congestion, "air cups," referred to in Islamic medicine as *Hujam,* are used. The air cups are made of glass, wide at the base and narrow at the top. After the hair in the intended area of treatment is shaved, a small piece of alcohol-soaked cotton is placed in the air cup and lighted; the cup is placed on the back (or problem area) of the sick person for 3 to 10 minutes. Several air cups are usually used at a time, with the intent to suck and direct the blood flow to the chest area by creating pressure. It is believed that by enhancing the blood flow to the chest area, chest congestion and persistent coughs will be relieved. In rare cases, after the cups are used, incisions are made in the area to release some of the sucked blood. This is done in cases of hypertension and in suspected cases of poisoning (Al-Refa'ai, 1990).

Fever is a cause for alarm and is usually treated by placing the sick person in bed with heavy covers. Children and babies are wrapped in blankets and made to "sweat out the fever." This is based on the belief that sweating will decrease the fever, if not eliminate it right away. Pharmaceutical reducing agents are also used concomitantly to reduce the fever, the most common of them aspirin.

Evil Eye, Envy (ein el hassad or el ein el wehshah). Another belief system that may explain health and illness states is the evil eye. Harfouche (1981) said that the fear of the evil eye influences the entire belief system of Middle Eastern people. There is a common belief among the people of the Middle East that the "evil eye puts the camel into the pot and mankind into the grave" (Donaldson, 1938, p. 66). People who are envious, often referred to as people with "empty-eye" or with a "blue eye," have the power to cause illness. Possessors of an evil eye may or may not know that they have it; thus the harm may be unintended. Such a person may be a neighbor, friend, relative, or a stranger (Donaldson, 1938; Harfouche, 1981).

People exert their "evil effect" by glaring and watching the person or the object and by speaking of the admired person or object in a boastful manner without mentioning the name of the God or the Cross (Harfouche, 1981). Infants are particularly susceptible and can become ill due to the evil eye. Tremors, convulsive seizures, severe spells of crying, refusal to nurse, and skin-color changes, such as pallor or blueness, have all been attributed to the evil eye. Nursing mothers may experience "drying up" or complete suppression of their milk. If the evil eye hits the breast, it becomes painful, swollen, and inflamed, or it may even develop a boil or abscess. The mother is incapacitated, her milk supply decreases or dries up completely, and her affected breast ceases to function (Harfouche, 1981). Evil eye results may be instantaneous; some claim that people have died immediately after exposure to a person who was envious of them and who may have given them the evil eye, but the power of the evil eye may also work slowly (Donaldson, 1938).

Various protective and therapeutic mechanisms are used to protect people against the evil eye. Preventive devices such as charms or amulets of blue beads or in shapes of the horseshoe or crescent are often used. Relics or religious charms, often referred to as *hijab* or *hirz* (that which is written and hidden to protect and fortify without being seen) are also used. Curative devices may involve seeking a *Raki* (traditional healer), who by resorting to supernatural forces, becomes endowed with the power of controlling or changing the course of an event. Purification of the environment with incense, along with prayers read over the head of the afflicted person, is another curative device used, among many others (Harfouche, 1981).

There are some indications that Arab Middle Eastern immigrants continue to value and practice some of these beliefs. However, despite these popular or folk beliefs, Arab Middle Eastern immigrants in the United States place a very high value on Western medicine, which epitomizes expertise, science, equipment, and consultants. Even though Arab Middle Eastern Americans continue to speak of the evil eye and the concepts of hot and cold as contributory factors in causing disease, Western medicine is sought after and practiced (Meleis, 1981).

Pregnancy and Motherhood

Reproductive behavior among Arab women in different Arab Middle Eastern countries has some common features. According to Omran (1980, p. 81), fertility is high, with childbearing starting early and continuing throughout the reproductive span. The age of marriage is generally low, and marriage is universal. The traditional preference is for sons and large families (Meleis, 1991). Fertility in the

Arab Middle East is still a major determinant of a wife's status in the family and community and a sign of virility for men. Arab Middle Eastern people tend to view children as economic and social assets, adding to the family's income and providing old-age security for the parents. Because of the high rate of infant mortality, which remains one of the highest in the world, only a small percentage of Arab couples use contraception regularly and efficiently (Omran, 1980, p. 82). Griffith (1982) said "nowhere in a culture are there usually more prescribed rituals and ways of behaving as are found surrounding childbearing and childrearing" (p. 81). In Middle Eastern countries, pregnancy improves the woman's status in the family, as well as in society (Meleis, 1991). As a result, women are expected to become pregnant as soon as they get married. Family members, especially on the husband's side, closely watch the newly married woman for signs of pregnancy. A mother's status is most secure if her first child is a boy.

A similar meaning of pregnancy is held in other developing countries. Among Haitian people, a pregnant woman gets more attention and help and is treated with more respect and pride (Dempsey & Gesse, 1983; Meleis & Aly, 1994). In Middle Eastern cultures, a pregnant woman is exempt from heavy housework. Other family members are expected to release women from some of the heavy daily chores. Craving is an acceptable and expected symptom of pregnancy, and it is the husband's responsibility to fulfill his wife's needs.

During labor, the husband may accompany his wife, together with other female family members. However, during delivery, the husband will usually wait outside while the wife's mother or other female family members stay with her. Middle Eastern men do not want to be pushed to participate in the delivery, and this does not negate the fact that they are very concerned about their wives (Meleis & Sorell, 1981).

Middle Easterners celebrate the newborn's first week of survival (*Saba'n or Sebu'*) through gatherings of family and friends. The rituals differ from one country to another. In some, seven different types of grains are soaked in water as a sign of fertile rich life just before the ceremony. The newborn wears a new, preferably white gown, and candles are lit as a sign of a bright future. If the parents can afford it, a sheep is sacrificed and distributed to poor people. Sometimes the sex of the newborn and the parents' sex preference influences the magnitude of the celebration. A boy's *Sebu'* is likely to be more extravagant than a girl's.

Middle Eastern women observe 40 days postpartum. During this period, they are pampered by their husbands and other family members. No sexual intercourse is allowed during this period for religious reasons; the woman is considered impure as long as she has vaginal bleeding. During the 40 days postpartum, the woman eats a hot, high-protein diet, with emphasis on chicken and meat.

Middle Eastern women are uncomfortable about praising their infants in the presence of strangers, to prevent the evil eye from causing any harm to them. Indochinese women use similar strategies to prevent the spirits from becoming jealous and taking away the newborn baby (Hollingsworth, Brown, & Brooten, 1980). Some Middle Easterners also believe that cutting the nails of newborn infants may bring some future harm to them, and therefore they may want to postpone that action for 40 days. The belief that cutting the newborn's nails may cause harm is also common among Indochinese eople, who believe that such action causes heart problems (Hollingsworth et al., 1980).

Middle Eastern women tend to breast-feed their babies for an average of 2 years. Some rely on this as a contraceptive method and may not seek birth-control consultation during the breast-feeding period. Unfortunately, bottle feeding was promoted in many countries, and artificial milk was distributed for free to substitute for breast feeding. Different types of food are believed to increase the breast-milk flow, and others are believed to cause health problems to the baby. *Halawa* (a sesame seed extract mixed with sugar), chicken soup, and *melokhia* (an Egyptian-grown, spinach-like vegetable eaten in a soup) belong to the first category, and citric fruit, garlic, and hot pepper belong to the second. There are no data to support or contradict any of these beliefs.

Perception of Symptoms

Arab Middle Eastern clients usually present generalized, more global, and less specific descriptions of their health and illness status.

Disease and trauma are thought to affect the individual as a whole. Mind and body are not separate; they are one and the same. A vague description of illness is also partly due to the lack of a framework that would permit careful description of signs and symptoms and their association with different parts of the body (Meleis, 1981).

Somatization is a pattern of expressing emotional symptoms. As in other Mediterranean and non-Western cultures, expression of anxiety, depression, and mental distress is likely to be in physical terms (Budman, Lipson, & Meleis, 1992). Physical complaints are a legitimate way of expressing personal and interpersonal problems. Consequently, the Arab patient with depression or anxiety commonly presents in outpatient medical settings with a variety of somatic complaints, such as diffuse pain, poor appetite, fatigue, or shortness of breath (Budman et al., 1992; El-Islam, 1982; Racy, 1980).

With regard to perception of pain, Arab Middle Easterners do not welcome painful experiences or suffering. They tend to show present-time orientation to pain and to focus on its immediacy. Although they tend to conceal outward expression of pain in the presence of strangers, under certain circumstances (such as labor and delivery pain), women's responses tend to be demonstrative, vigorous, and public. In fact, cultural norms not only permit loud moans, groans, and screams but also expect it (Reizian & Meleis, 1986).

Among the few studies that focused on Arab Middle Eastern immigrants is one conducted by Reizian and Meleis (1987) to identify patterns of medical complaints among Arab Middle Eastern patients in the United States. Their sample included 102 immigrants from several Arab Middle Eastern countries, including Palestine, Jordan, Yemen, Lebanon, Saudi Arabia, Iraq, Egypt, and Kuwait. Using the Arabic version of the *Cornell Medical Index,* the authors found that most complaints were related to the digestive system and the cardiovascular system; symptoms related to level of sensitivity and to a sense of inadequacy. Next in frequency were the respiratory system and the genitourinary system; symptoms related to the level of fatigability and frequency of illness. The authors also found that increased age was significantly correlated with all symptoms, level of education was negatively correlated with all symptoms, and religion, sex, and marital status were not related to symptom patterns. The country of origin of research participants was significantly related to patterns of perceived symptomatology, with Palestinians and

Jordanians reporting more physical-biological symptoms than Lebanese, Iraqis, and Egyptians. Occupational status also was related to patterns of perceived symptoms, with the unemployed reporting significantly higher scores on symptoms representing physical-biological systems.

In another study, Iraqi American refugees were compared to refugees from Poland, Romania, and Vietnam (Young, Bukoff, Waller, & Blount, 1987). Compared to the other three refugee groups, Iraqis tended to rate their global health as equally favorable, but they were the least likely to rate their mental health negatively. This is a significant finding, considering that 62% of the Iraqis indicated they have at least seven mental health symptoms and that they were more than twice as likely as any other group to report physical complaints, most of them involving gastrointestinal, skin, ear, nose, and throat problem and feelings of dizziness. Dental health was rated the least favorable among the four groups but more significantly so among the Iraqis (poor dental health ranged from 3% of the Romanians to 39% of the Iraqis). No menstrual problems were reported among Iraqi women. (The authors attributed this to their cultural resistance to discussing gynecological problems, rather than to the absence of symptoms.) The overwhelming majority of Iraqi refugee women (71%) delivered their babies at home. Also, although 80% of the Iraqis reported using a physician's office for health care, Iraqis also reported the highest incidence of untreated health problems (74% reported one or more untreated health problems). They singled out the doctor-patient relationship and understanding and transportation as most troublesome in receiving and accessing the care they need.

These studies, along with the population study of the Arab Middle Eastern countries, provide many insights on health patterns and health problems Arab Middle Eastern immigrant women might encounter, but given the lack of the specific focus on women, generalizations of these findings are problematic, and the findings should be interpreted with caution.

Coping Strategies

When health professionals work with Middle Eastern immigrant women, they need to know how these women tend to deal with illness, stress, or crisis in their lives or in the lives of their families. Arab Middle Eastern immigrant women tend to use strategies that enhance harmony and minimize conflict. Conceptualizations and synthesis of the various coping strategies used by Arab Middle Eastern immigrant women has led to identifying and formulating two prominent and major coping strategies. These coping strategies are identified as power (familial and structural alliances) and roles (accommodating and confronting) (Meleis, 1993).

POWER: FAMILIAL AND STRUCTURAL ALLIANCES

Arab women's power is poorly understood, because of the absence of symbols that are more familiar within a Western framework. Modest clothes, covered hair, evasive eyes, silent responses, and accepting demeanor are all considered symbols of disempowerment in the West. Homemaking roles, limited decision making in front of strangers, and deferral to other members of the family are interpreted by health care professionals as representing lack of power. Although these manifestations may represent lack of power in some situations, to the discriminating eye and the culturally informed, these manifestations may also represent temporary deferral of expectations and cultural rituals of role play. Arab women in the United States use strategies they used in their country of origin; they derive their power and status in the family through developing family alliances. There is support in the literature for the view that Arab women's power increases with age, with having sons, and with forming an alliance with in-laws and/or elders in their family. The elderly in these alliances support women's decisions and give credence to women's voices. Similarly, having grown-up sons and daughters also gives women stronger voices.

Some changes have occurred, however, in the source of alliances and support for Arab immigrant women. Many immigrant women have no access to wise and elderly relatives, nor to sons and daughters. Some women expressed concern that their Americanized sons and daughters refuse to play the mediator and supporter role. Others expected health care professionals to play the role of intermediary. The extent to which women are able to restructure their power base determines their power and status. Those who were able to develop new alliances based in health care systems and other institutions, such as schools, social clubs, or other community groups, were able to slowly develop a new power base that supports their decision. These alliances empowered them to cope with illness, stress, and crises. Health care professionals can uncover these resources, and they usually are able to effect change, promote self-care, and increase adherence to health promotion behaviors.

ROLES: ACCOMMODATING AND CONFRONTING

Westerners value a confrontational approach to dealing with diagnosis, illness management, and health promotion. Moreover, health care professionals also expect their clients to deal with health and illness issues straightforwardly and forthrightly. When clients present a more reflective "wait and see" or "do for me what you should," clients are labeled difficult, uninterested, or refusing to take responsibility for their own lives. Middle Eastern women tend to cope with new and difficult situations by making accommodations. They are socialized as negotiators, integrators, buffers, and caregivers. To expect them to meet a challenging parenting crisis, a grave diagnosis, or a challenging procedure by confronting it creates stress and is counterproductive. Immigrant patients may prefer to be told in stages and small doses about the gravity of a diagnosis rather than all at once and in great detail. They also play many hidden roles that may interfere with their clinic appointments. Like other marginalized groups, they are in an "in between position" (Hall, Stevens, & Meleis, 1994). They are negotiators and buffers among and between spouses, in-laws, institutions, host communities, and home communities (Meleis & Rogers, 1987). They work hard at balancing all the values that different entities represent, and they work at integrating and maintaining country-of-origin values and belief systems. As a result, they may experience role overload, marital stress, discipline problems, and nutritional deprivation (Hattar-Pollara & Meleis, 1995). Some may cope by becoming depressed and present themselves to the health care system with somatic complaints. They find themselves in a health care system that lacks culturally competent care due to language, lack of understanding of stressors, racism, politicism, or stereotyping, and they may not have access to it due to lack of transportation or role overload.

Use of Health Resources

Full or appropriate use of health resources by immigrant women in the United States is often constrained by a number of factors. Women immigrants carry along with them their own conception and understanding of health services, and on the basis of such understanding, they approach and seek health services according to the patterns they were accustomed to in their country of origin. The complexity of U.S. health care services and frequency of system changes are other factors that complicate their efforts to acquire familiarity with the system and achieve the needed working knowledge and understanding of health resources. In addition, language and cultural barriers, transportation, role overload, and confrontations between their own versus health providers' expectations of self-care are often grounds for much of the confusion, misunderstanding, and dissatisfactions on both parts.

To pinpoint the issues faced by Arab Middle Eastern immigrant women in their use of health resources, it is important to understand their own framework of health care. The health care system of Arab countries in the Middle East is very different from the U.S. system. One feature of the Arab Middle East system is that health care is viewed as the primary responsibility of the government, and it is often provided free of charge. Specific services, such as school health services, maternal health services, worker health services, and public health services, are administered by corresponding governmental bodies and ministries (Omran, 1980). Access to and use of these health services are mostly dependent on the consumers' health needs. These services are understood to be geared to curing rather than preventive care. On the basis of what they were accustomed to, Arab Middle Eastern immigrant women generally face numerous difficulties in accessing the appropriate U.S. health care resources.

Not having a clear picture of the mechanics and the value structure of the American health care system, Arab Middle Eastern immigrant women may end up using the wrong resources. Generally they depend on word of mouth about who is good, and they may end up moving from one provider to another until they find the care and reciprocity they need. From the viewpoint of the health care provider, however, failure to establish a consistent relationship and failure to seek preventive health care, as in the case of preparing for childbirth, are looked down upon, with subsequent distress for the client.

Private health insurance has been, until recently, a foreign concept for the people of the Arab Middle East. Thus, except for the affluent or the fully employed, immigrant Arab Middle Eastern women generally do not subscribe to health insurance. Those who own businesses prefer to pay for treatment of illnesses rather than paying the high monthly insurance premiums. The complexity of procedures for insurance reimbursement, coupled with distrust of insurance, are reasons behind the refusal to purchase health insurance. Administrators of health care facilities usually disregard or devalue clients without health insurance.

Arab Middle Eastern immigrant women tend to face numerous roadblocks set up by hospital administrators to guarantee payment before they actually get treated. Also, in the Arab Middle East, and in some European and non-Western countries, many people use pharmacists for symptomatic treatment of illnesses, in lieu of physicians. Clients describe their symptoms or simply request a certain medication without a prescription. Because of the high cost of medication in the United States or their frustration with the system, some Arab Americans seek to acquire medication from their countries of origin.

Certain norms and cultural values may influence patterns of interaction with the U.S. health care system. Although Arab Middle Eastern immigrant women display a great respect for Western medicine, they also tend to relate competence to the power base of health care providers. Higher-ranking health care providers are accorded more trust and confidence. Thus, their satisfaction with the care they receive depends on who, in their perception, is providing the care (Meleis, 1981).

Modesty is another cultural value that influences interaction. Their embarrassment in discussing female disorders and symptoms associated with female genitourinary systems with male health care providers forces Arab Middle Eastern immigrant women to seek female physicians or nurses rather than health providers of the opposite sex (Racy, 1980).

Generally, the health-seeking behavior of Arab Middle Easterners, except for the socioeconomically advantaged, is limited to curative rather than preventive treatment. Hospitalizations are feared "because hospitals are considered places of misfortune where people go to die" (Lipson & Meleis, 1983, p. 857). The dependent sick role is assumed when an Arab Middle Easterner becomes ill. The patient is usually exempted from all role responsibilities and is cared for by members of the immediate and/or extended family. Social obligations during times of illness dictate frequent visits, along with gifts of home-cooked meals to the hospital or the home of the sick person. These social and cultural attributes are often misunderstood by health care providers and consequently incorrectly managed. The outcome may lead to further alienation and more barriers to accessing the appropriate health resources.

Magnusson & Aurelius (1980) observed that immigrants overuse the emergency rooms. Similar observations were reported about Arab clients in the health care system. However, a medical record review study on Arab American patients did not substantiate this observation (Lipson et al., 1987). It is probable, however, that recent immigrants who lack the social network or the know-how to access health resources may resort to emergency rooms for lack of other avenues.

Conclusions

Arab American women have received very little attention in recent literature. Although they are appearing in increasing numbers in the health care system, attempts to understand them are very scarce. The available literature attests to the fact that Middle Eastern immigrant women are among the least studied ethnic groups. There is a serious lack of studies that focus on different aspects of the Middle Eastern immigrant woman's life, her role in the immigration process, the changes she experiences as a result of immigration, what problems she encounters in the new land, and what are her coping styles.

The previous review points out some of the gaps that need to be considered if this population is to be understood and ultimately helped. Research needs to be conducted in such areas as women's roles and status before and after migration to the United States; change in support systems upon migration and their effect on immigrant women; and health beliefs and practices, whether or not they change upon migration, and to what extent. The problems Middle Eastern immigrant women may face in the new environment are usually due to the language barrier and unfamiliarity with the system. This is probably true for most non-English speaking immigrants as well.

The intent of this chapter was to provide a framework that may enhance understanding of the situation of Arab Middle Eastern immigrants. Health care professionals may use the content with caution. Ultimately, the diversity among this population, as well as their immigration history and experiences, will determine the response to health and illness and will profoundly influence outcomes.

References

Abraham, S. (1983). Detroit's Arab-American community: A survey of diversity and commonality. In S. S. Abraham & N. N. Abraham (Eds.), *Arabs in the new world* (pp. 85-108). Michigan: Wayne State University.

Al-Refa'ai, M. D. (1990). *Al-tadawi bil-hujama fil Islam* [Pressure-suction treatment in Islam]. Jordan: Collaborating Publishing Co.

Budman, C. L., Lipson, J. G., & Meleis, A. I. (1992). The cultural consultant in mental health care: The case of an Arab adolescent. *American Journal of Orthopsychiatry, 62*(3), 359-370.

Dempsey, P. A., & Gesse, T. (1983, May-June). The childbearing Haitian refugee—Cultural applications to clinical nursing. *Public Health Reports, 98*(3), 261-267.

Donaldson, B. A. (1938). *The wild rue: A study of Muhammadan magic and folklore in Iran.* London: Luzac.

Carrier, R. L. (1966). The hot-cold syndrome and symbolic balance in Mexican and Spanish-American folk medicine. *Ethnology, 5,* 251-263.

Elkholy, A. (1969). The Arab Americans: Nationalism and traditional preservations. In E. C. Hasopian & A. Paden (Eds.), *Studies in assimilation* (pp. 3-17). Illinois: The Medina University Press International.

El-Islam, M. (1982). Overview: Arabic cultural psychiatry. *Transcultural Psychiatric Research Review, 19,* 5-24.

Fouad, N. (1986). *Family planning behavior of Arab-American women.* Unpublished doctoral dissertation, University of California, San Francisco, School of Nursing.

Griffith, S. (1982, May/June). Childbearing and the concept of culture. *Journal of Gynecological Nursing,* 181-184.

Haddad, Y. (1983). Arab Muslims and Islamic institutions in America: Adaptation and reform. In S. S. Abraham & N. N. Abraham (Ed.), *Arabs in the new world* (pp. 65-81). Michigan: Wayne State University.

Hall, J. M., Stevens, P. E., & Meleis, A. I. (1994). Marginalization: A guiding concept for valuing diversity in nursing knowledge development. *Advances in Nursing Science, 16*(4), 23-41.

Harfouche, J. K. (1981). The evil eye and infant health in Lebanon. In A. Dundes (Ed.), *The evil eye: A folklore casebook* (pp. 86-106). New York: Garland.

Hattar-Pollara, M., & Meleis, A. I. (in press). *The daily lived experiences of Jordanian immigrant women in the U.S.: Stress of immigrants.*

Hattar-Pollara, M., & Meleis, A. I. (1995). Parenting adolescents: Jordanian immigrant women in California. *Health Care for Women International, 16,* 195-211.

Hollingsworth, A. O., Brown, L. P., & Brooten, A. A. (1980, November). The refugees and childbearing: What to expect. *RN,* 45-48.

Lipson, J. G., & Meleis, A. I. (1983). Issues in health care of Middle Eastern patients. *Western Journal of Medicine, 139,* 854.

Lipson, J. G., Reizian, A., & Meleis, A. I. (1987). Arab-American patients: A medical record review. *Social Science and Medicine, 24*(2), 101-107.

Madsen, W. (1955). Hot and cold in the universe of San Francisco Tescospa Valley of Mexico. *Journal of American Folklore, 68,* 123-139.

Magnusson, G., & Aurelius, G. (1980). Illness behavior and nationality. *Social Science and Medicine, 14A,* 357.

May, K. M. (1992). Middle-Eastern immigrant parents—Social network and help-seeking for child health care. *Journal of Advanced Nursing, 17,* 905-912.

Mehdi, B. T. (1978). *The Arabs in America: 1492-1977.* New York: Oceana Publication, Inc., Dobbs and Ferry.

Meleis, A. I. (1981). The Arab American in the Western health care system. *American Journal of Nursing, 6,* 1180-1183.

Meleis, A. I. (1991). Between two cultures: Identity, roles, and health. *Health Care for Women International, 12,* 365-377.

Meleis, A. I. (1993, June 25-28). *Being a Middle Eastern immigrant in the U.S: Triumphs and tribulations.* Paper presented at ICN's symposium on Immigration/Refugee Experiences: Women as Immigrants and Refugees, Madrid.

Meleis, A. I., & Aly, F. (1994). Women's health: A global perspective. In J. McCloskey & H. Grance (Eds.), *Current issues in nursing* (4th ed., pp. 1992-1993). New York: C. V. Mosby (Mosby Year Book).

Meleis, A. I., Dallafar, A., & Lipson, J. G. (1995). *The reluctant immigrant: Immigration experiences among Middle Eastern immigrant groups in northern California.* Manuscript submitted for publication.

Meleis, A. I., & Rogers, S. (1987). Women in transition: Being vs. becoming or being and becoming. *Health Care for Women International, 8,* 199-217.

Meleis, A. I., & Sorell, L. (1981). The Arab American women and their birth experience. *The American Journal of Maternal Child Nursing, 6,* 171-176.

Naff, A. (1980). Arabs. In S. Therstrom (Ed.), *Harvard encyclopedia of American ethnic groups* (pp. 128-136). Cambridge, MA: Harvard University Press.

Naff, A. (1983). Arabs in America: A historical overview. In S. S. Abraham & N. N. Abraham (Eds.), *Arabs in the new world* (pp. 9-29). Michigan: Wayne State University.

Nigem, E. (1986). Arab Americans: Migrations, socioeconomic and demographic characteristics. *International Migration Review, 20*(3), 629-645.

Omran, A. (1980). *Population in the Arab world.* New York: United Nations Fund for Population Activities & Eroom Helm Ltd.

Pessar, P. R. (1984). The linkage between the household and workplace of Dominican women in the U.S. *IMR, 18*(4), 1188-1211.

Pliskin, K. (1992). Dysphoria and somatization in Iranian culture. *Western Journal of Medicine, 9*(57), 295-300.

Racy, J. (1980). Somatization in Saudi women: A therapeutic challenge. *British Journal of Psychiatry, 137*, 212-216.

Ragucci, A. (1981). Italian Americans. In A. Harwood (Ed.), *Ethnicity and medical care* (pp. 211-263). Cambridge, MA: Harvard University Press.

Reizian, A., & Meleis, A. I. (1986). Arab-Americans' perceptions of and response to pain. *Critical Care Nurse, 6*(6), 30-37.

Reizian, A., & Meleis, A. I. (1987). Symptoms reported by Arab-American patients on the Cornell Medical Index. *Western Journal of Nursing Research, 9*(3), 368-384.

U.S. Bureau of the Census. (1979). *Ancestry of the population* (Current population survey). Washington, DC: Government Printing Office.

U.S. Bureau of the Census. (1980). *Ancestry of the population* (Current population survey). Washington, DC: Government Printing Office.

U.S. Bureau of the Census. (1990). *Ancestry of the population by country of origin.* Berkeley: University of California CD-ROM Information System, Lawrence Berkeley Laboratory.

U.S. Bureau of the Census. (1992). *Population by race.* Washington, DC: Government Printing Office.

Wasfi, A. (1971). *An Islamic-Lebanese community in the U.S.A.: A study in cultural anthropology.* Beirut: Beirut Arab University.

Wigle, L., & Abraham, S. (1974). Arab nationalism in America: The Dearborn Arab community. In D. W. Hartman (Ed.), *Immigrants and migrants: The Detroit ethnic experience* (pp. 279-302). Detroit: New University Thought Publishing Co.

Young, R. F., Bukoff, A., Waller, J. B., & Blount, S. B. (1987). Health status, health problems, and practices among refugees from the Middle East, Eastern Europe, and Southeast Asia. *International Migration Review, 21*(3), 760-782.

Younis, A. (1961). *The coming of the Arabic-speaking people to the United States.* Unpublished PhD dissertation, Boston University.

10 Health Care on the Inside

CHRISTINE JOSE-KAMPFNER

Fourteen years ago, I took a job as a counselor in a Midwest women's prison. This experience changed the way that I think about "women's" issues. Suddenly, a hidden population of women became visible to me. Like most Americans, men and women in prison have always occupied an unconscious part of my imagination. In fact, they were central to the way that I understood *good* and *bad*, *morality*, and *corruptness*. In my imagination, prisons confined the socially unacceptable to an invisible yet important place. They were locked up in jail, out of sight. My identity was dependent on this imaginary, invisible and criminal population because they justified my goodness, my morality, in comparison to their badness and immorality. This dichotomy also informed the goodness and morality of the imagined society always in the process of cleansing itself of "bad" elements.

When I began to work with women in prison, these dichotomies fell apart. I understood that in fact women in prison are just that. They are women who are in prison. They are not first "prisoners" or "criminals." These women are not corrupt or immoral. Most of them serve short sentences for petty crimes. Furthermore, they do not disappear into the depths of prison. They move out of the criminal justice system and are outsiders again after their terms are over.

Although all of this research was conducted in prisons, it is worth noting that women's health care in jails is even worse than what is provided in prison. Jails hold approximately 3.4 million people annually, approximately 35 times the number of people handled by all state and federal prisons. Women's experiences in jails are quite different from their experiences in prison. In most jails, women are housed in the same building as men, but intermingling between the sexes is almost never permitted. (This effective limit of heterosociability serves as one form of punishment for criminality. It metaphorically cuts off inmates from socially legitimate forms of sexuality.) Many wardens thus keep women locked in their cells while men circulate, and vice versa. However, because the male population in prison is generally much larger than the female population, many wardens simply keep women locked in their cells for a significant part of their day. For example, in Michigan jails, women are permitted to leave their cells only for meals and on Wednesday afternoons, whereas men are allowed to circulate the other 6 days of the week. The justification for these decisions is based on racist and sexist assumptions about the behavior of male and female criminals. Wardens assume that men, most of whom are men of color, will become violent if they are held under lock and key too long. Conversely, it is assumed that women in prison, most of whom are also of color, will become more complacent. This kind of treatment compounds the difficulties of women in jail. Usually, this is the most difficult time for women in the criminal justice system. It is the beginning of their separation from their children, their loved ones, and the outside. At the same time, their future is constantly unsure. A consensus among the women whom I interviewed was clearly stated by one inmate: "The hardest time you ever do is while you are waiting in jail."

The kind of reasoning that leads to this conclusion—racist, sexist, and generally uncaring of the humanity of incarcerated people—unfortunately informs the decisions of too many administrators and guards in the prison and jail system. As I will demonstrate, incarcerated women, a preponderance of whom are of color, suffer from the worst health care in the United States; their living environment regularly challenges their ability to maintain good health. These injustices cannot be overlooked in any evaluation of the state of women's health in this country.

I have met women who lost their battles against a system that assigns them to positions of impoverishment and maintains their marginality by committing them to prison. It was striking to see that so many of the women in prison were women of color. These are compounded statistics and may vary by region, but they reflect a large general trend that is consistent across the nation. I saw myself in their eyes. I understood that we were not so different, that we shared values and hopes, fears and dreams. But one significant difference separated me from them. That difference was socioeconomic. About 72% of women in prison were unemployed at the time of their arrest. The overwhelming similarity among all of these criminal women was that on the outside, most of them had been living in or near poverty. These criminals were women who had been struggling to survive. I found women who had written bad checks in order to support their children, women who had killed their abusive spouses in self-defense, women who had stolen, women who had been sexually abused, and women who took drugs to ease the pain of their lives. About 72% of the crimes committed by women in prison are victimless crimes. About 32.8% of women in jail are there on drug charges, and 35% were convicted of property crimes.

The vast majority of women in prison had limited access to resources on the outside. It quickly became apparent that they were denied these same resources when they lived behind bars.

Women in prison are overwhelmingly of color. Latina and African American women make up 72% of the female prison population in Michigan, a state in which less than 20% of all women are Latina and African American. Historically, women of color have been over-represented in correctional populations. In 1980, when Black women made up 14% of the female U.S. population, they accounted for nearly half of the total female prison population (Michigan Women's Commission, 1987). Although equal numbers of white women and women of color are arrested, women of color account for more than 50% of prison populations nationwide. Women of color are over-represented in the criminal justice system, and they consistently receive harsher treatment in the hands of the court. White women are far more likely to receive probationary sentences or to have their charges dismissed than are non-white women. This is even more common in crimes that are frequently committed by women, such as larceny, forgery, and fraud. These statistics are not incidental to an understanding of women in prison. Indeed, they are central. Men and women of color are treated as threats to (white) American citizens, rather than as citizens themselves.

As I became more familiar with prison life, I realized that on the inside, women prisoners continued to have inadequate access to resources. Before they came to prison, most of them were poor and did not receive adequate health care. Once inside prison, they became criminals and were once again denied health care. The state neglects the minds and bodies of an "undeserving" population. Prisons are reflections of a society where sexism, racism, and classism deny adequate health care to women of color and to poor women of all races.

Gender stereotyping has especially affected the handling of women at all stages of prison development. In the 19th century, women were commonly regarded as more immoral than men; as a corollary, criminal females were more depraved than males and hence less deserving (Rafter, 1985). This has important implications. The health of women in prisons has been neglected. Their complaints are often dismissed as "psychosomatic" problems. Women's health concerns were not taken seriously in the 19th century or today.

It is important to consider the historical context from which these issues of health and prison were derived. Michel Foucault's *Discipline and Punish: The Birth of the Prison* offers an understanding of how, in modern times, the body is used as an avenue to the souls of prisoners. He explains that the contemporary criminal justice system is predicated on the assumption that it is more civilized than the barbarity of preenlightened Europe. "Enlightened" prison reformers saw themselves as advocates for prisoners. They ostensibly attempted to humanize the criminal justice system.

But, Foucault explains, the new system is equally dependent on absolute control. In the past, offenders were forced to bear their punishments on their bodies with branding, so that they would permanently display the marks of their shame and powerlessness. Now, punishment is less focused on physical pain and instead favors humiliation through psychological control. "The expiation that once rained down upon the body [has been] replaced by a punishment that acts in depth on the heart, the thoughts, the will, and the inclinations" (Foucault, 1979, p. 16).

Although Foucault bases his arguments on what happens to the body, he does not discuss the body as gendered or racialized. The experiences of torture and control are influenced by the ways that people understood their bodies before they entered the criminal justice system. Thus, women's issues of control, including an investigation of sexual abuse, must be a part of an investigation of the experiences of women's health in prison.

Health Care in Prison

According to the Federal Bureau of Prisons, 62,256 women were incarcerated in state and federal prisons in 1994 (this figure does not include women in jails). Of these, 55,365 women were in state prisons and 6,891 are in federal prisons. A disproportionate number of women come from a minority group: 46% are African American, 22.7% are Latina, 5.5% are Asian American, and 25.8% are white. These numbers combine state and federal statistics.

The major concentration of African American women in prison is in the South, with 10,256 Black women in prison, and in the Midwest, with approximately 3,500 African American women in prison. Before their imprisonment, 73% were unemployed; 66.3% were between 18 and 34 years old, and 25.5% were between 35 and 44 years old; 82% were mothers; and 60% had not finished high school.

This chapter is an effort to examine the health care and health of Latina and African American women in prison through the larger project of an exploration of health care for all women in prison. Health care is an enormous issue for women in prison because it is so intimately related to power and control, which are central concerns for women in prison. The women in prison whom we interviewed were extremely preoccupied with their bodies. They explained that their physical well-being became an enormous worry because of their lack of control over their bodies as a result of incarceration and the denial of adequate health care in prison. Dying in prison was one of their worst fears, because it symbolized defeat in the face of the controlling system. One woman expressed these concerns:

With the constant strip searches, the cells, the constant restriction of movement, I am always kept aware of the fact that my body's not mine. . . . They take everything away from you. Your family, your friends, your life, and even the control over what you can do about your goddam period!

Prisons are concerned with the control, containment, and isolation of people who are labeled criminal, not with their health. Thus, prison guards and wardens stress obedience, conformity, and passivity. They do not pay attention to the needs of women prisoners but instead cultivate an environment that facilitates watching and controlling their movement.

Correctional institutions wield enormous power over the bodies of incarcerated women. Unfortunately, health care is not a central part of this regimen. Control of their bodies supersedes "upkeep." One prisoner explained, "They aren't in the business of keeping us fit and healthy, they are in the business of keeping us locked up." Thus, women do not receive regular checkups. The only medical examination that is a part of prison routine is a yearly gynecological exam, and even that is often not administered.

Nurses are responsible for the majority of health care services in most prisons. Unfortunately, the scope of their practice is "illness care," focused on crisis management and the administration of medicine. Preventive medicine is rarely part of the repertoire in prisons. Thus, preventable problems and diseases receive attention only after women are already sick. This contributes to the preventable spread of viruses and to more damaging bouts of illness. Thus, women in prison receive the same kind of health care that they might find in hospital emergency rooms, on which many relied before their terms. Physicians are usually available in nearby hospitals. The prison setting lacks appropriate facilities for professional practice.

The lack of health care in prisons is merely an exaggerated version of the already poor care that most of these inmates had on the outside. The vast majority of incarcerated women come from impoverished communities; more often than not, they have been living below the poverty line before their arrests. A poverty-line access to resources is maintained once these women are put behind bars. Sexual and emotional abuse, as familiar as poverty before incarceration, continue to be part of their lives behind prison walls.

The disadvantages that prisoners faced on the outside of prison do not go away once they are brought through the prison gates. On the outside, Latinos suffer from a higher rate of poverty than any other racial or ethnic group in the United States, even though their rate of employment is higher than that of African Americans. More than one fourth of all Latinos and African Americans in the United States live in poverty, and this proportion is probably greater for Latinas. Furthermore, they have the lowest rate of insurance on the outside. Although these problems are often based on illegal immigration into this country, the vast majority of Latinos were born in the United States. For example, 68% of Mexican Americans living in the United States were also born in this country, and many have been here for many generations (U.S. Office of the Surgeon General, 1993).

Women's health in prison depends on the willingness of the institution's representatives to acknowledge that they actually need health care, something that sounds easy but in fact becomes quite difficult for women in prison. As prisoners, women are infantilized. Their complaints are often ignored by guards, and without the guards, they have no access to medical care. Even when they do have access to medical care, health care personnel have been desensitized to the constant requests of "complaining" inmates, view inmates who seek care as manipulative, and usually minimize or ignore their complaints.

Prison Conditions

The loss of control that women experience in prison adversely affects their mental and physical health. Women who were adults on the outside are treated as children in prison. This humiliating circumstance complicates not only their health but their access to health care. In order to access health care, they must report their complaint to a prison guard, just as a child reports her pains to a parent. Thus, metaphorically, their medical complaints have to be heard by an "adult." The guards then decide if a woman's complaint actually merits attention, just as a parent decides for his or her child. This infantilization makes it almost impossible for women to take care of themselves. Some prison guards are sympathetic to the needs of women prisoners, but others are not. Women in prison, however, cannot control the attitudes or prejudices of their surrogate caretakers. When they are not taken seriously, their health is put in jeopardy, and they cannot do anything about it.

An example that illustrates the extent of this childlike position is menstruation. Women are regularly "disbelieved" when they get their periods. Like every part of their prison lives, the inconsistencies are pronounced and painful. When an inmate needs napkins, she is required to ask the guard for her monthly supply. If this is inadequate, she often needs a note from the nurse stating her further need. Some months a woman will have no problem acquiring sanitary napkins; other times, she might have to plead with a guard. This inconsistency itself is very difficult, because women cannot rely on their surroundings. Thus, they cannot create strategies to resist or even cope with the rules of the prison because the rules themselves change, depending on who administers them. Like children, these women can rely only on their capacity to be polite in the face of inconsistent adults. This uncontrollability itself causes depression.

Catherine: Prison is a place where women are treated as minor disobedient children. They are talked down to as children. Your work classification is often based on your ability to obey without questioning the smallest of rules.

Nora: Prison is where you are treated like a child and told to act like a woman. When you remind those in authority that you are not a child and you do not appreciate being treated as such, you are written up for an insubordinate behavior. If you maintain your individuality as a woman, you are labeled a troublemaker. On the other hand, if you give up your individuality, scratch your skin, grin, and become docile, you are well-behaved.

Women interviewed in prison report that when they go to the nurse feeling sick, they often leave with a diagnosis of psychosomatic illness. The tendency to dismiss women prisoners' complaints as psychosomatic is a reflection of the outside medical view that slips easily from *physically sick* to *mentally ill* for women. In classical psychoanalytic theory, there is no such a thing as a *mentally well* woman: The ambitious woman can be blamed for "emasculating" men, and the devoted mother can be blamed for "infecting" her sons with guilt and dependency.

We cannot rule out the possibility that many women in prison, like women on the outside, use sickness as an escape from their oppression as workers and mothers. They are not being dishonest or faking. Our culture encourages people to express resistance as illness, just as it encourages us to view overt rebellion as sick. The oppression is real; the resistance is real; but the sickness is manufactured.

Prison Life

Like women on the outside, women in prison experience depression, a complex psychological reaction to the stress of prison. A significant component of this stress is the lack of control that women in prison have over their bodies and their lives. Waites (1993) argued that the amount of control a woman has over her life is inversely related to the stress she experiences.

Sue: Prison life is such a sense of loss. Yes, of loss, you lose everything . . . even you.

Barbara: The real prison is a loneliness that sinks its teeth into your soul. It's an emptiness which leaves a sick feeling inside.

The women describe prison life as unreal. Life in prison is happening, but you cannot allow yourself to believe it is happening.

Catherine: I have been incarcerated for 10 years. Prison life has made me lose my memory. I used to have such a good memory, but now I do not even remember where I put things in my tiny little room. Your routine is the same. Your memories of this place you don't want to keep, so you don't have any memories. You never see any buildings or any flowers around here. It is hard to imagine the outside world. Everything is here in one level. There are no stairs, so you forget what it is like to go upstairs and downstairs. I remember one time that I had to go to court and they took my to this building in a big town. I felt lost, scared. The building looked huge. I felt dizzy. I forgot about the sound of the cars and the horns beeping. The everyday life sounds are nonexistent here.

Sally: In my opinion, prison is a very lonely place. It is a world within itself, indeed, a world that leaves one feeling empty inside and void of any real emotions.

Upon admission, the women are stripped of their personal property, their roles in the world, and most important of all, their pride. Roles such as mother, wife, prostitute—whatever gave meaning to the women's lives—are taken away, along with most of what personalized them on the outside. Their possessions are pawed and fingered by officials who itemize and prepare them for storage. The admission process is a violation of the body. The inmate herself may be frisked, and the search may include a rectal examination.

A prisoner: You know what your life in jail is going to be like the day you get admitted. From that day on, you are nobody. You are a number. You are stripped of your personal property and identification. Even your body is taken away. They can search you any time they please, including body cavities.

Prisoners cannot prevent staff and visitors from seeing them under these humiliating circumstances. The women are never free from exposure.

A prisoner: Prisoners are considered like property. We even have a code number. You are not Smith, but Number 34568. You know, being in jail is being out of your existence.

Women's Health Needs

Women prisoners' special health needs are often ignored. They need a different type of health care service than male offenders do. Women are not offered routine gynecological exams, routine breast assessment, health education, or services related to childbearing. The institutions that hold women's bodies do not pay attention to the fact that, as a result of their poverty and lack of health care, these women are at high risk for obstetrical problems, as they were even before they come to prison. The leading cause of death for all women aged

22 to 44 is breast cancer, and without breast examinations, avoidable cancer becomes lethal for women in prison (McGaha, 1986). For Latinas, diabetes presents a particular problem because it is common among this population. It is difficult for women to maintain the correct diet in prisons, and many have complained that guards and cooks disregard their needs. African American women have a high risk of cervical cancer, more than twice that of the white population, and their mortality rate from this disease is three times higher. Women in prison and jails often suffer from chronic heath concerns that go undiagnosed. These problems often develop as a result of a lifetime of poor nutrition and poor preventive care. From rotting teeth to venereal disease, their existing health problems become barriers to rehabilitation.

Although no specific study has been done with women, we know that approximately 1.2 million inmates in U.S. correctional institutions have a high prevalence of communicable diseases, such as human immunodeficiency virus (HIV) infection, tuberculosis, hepatitis B virus infection, and gonorrhea. Before their incarceration, the limited access to health care that most women in prison experience made it difficult to identify and treat them in the general community. Because of high yearly turnover (approximately 800% and 50% in jails and prisons, respectively), the criminal justice system can play an important public health role, both during incarceration and in the immediate postrelease period. A public policy agenda for criminal justice should include an epidemiologic orientation, as well as resources for education, counseling, early detection, and treatment (Glaser & Greifinger, 1993).

The treatment of pregnant women makes clear the system's lack of understanding of women's needs. Women in one Midwest prison are chained before being taken to give birth, with a guard accompanying them to delivery and recovery—as if they were likely to escape during labor or while delivering. The mothers are taken back to the prison within 24 hours after delivery, and the babies are placed with relatives or a department of social services.

It is difficult for women in prison to maintain a healthy and appropriate diet when they are pregnant. Women who are pregnant in prison are also at high risk for problems related to their emotional health. They are deprived of the kinds of emotional support ˍ depended on outside. Latina women particularly miss the special care that they received from their extended family network, which has traditionally valued and taken care of pregnant women.

Most efforts to improve medical conditions in these institutions have been mandated by the courts. For instance, as a result of lawsuits women prisoners and outside advocates have brought against prisons in Michigan, women prisoners are entitled to a yearly gynecological exam. However, the institutional bureaucracy is not required to provide any verification that the women have actually received exams; their word is accepted as true. As a result, women still find it difficult to register complaints and get their needs met.

Abuse

Most women come into prison with a history of physical or sexual abuse. By some estimates, as many as 90% of female prisoners were sexually abused before they came to prison. In prison, they are constantly forced to relive the trauma of violation of their bodies when subjected to body searches by male or female guards. An inmate must submit to a shakedown from a male or female guard at any time of the day or night. This involves standing at attention while a guard passes his or her hands all over the woman's body. The inmates talk about the helplessness and humiliation they feel in the face of the male guards, some of whom delight in giving a sharp chop to the women's crotch. As Barbara Deming (1966) described in *Prison Notes*,

> They wouldn't be able to admit it to themselves, but their search, of course, is for something else, and is efficient: their search is for our pride. And I think with a sinking heart, again and again, it must be, they find it and take it. (p. 4)

Some women report symptoms associated with posttraumatic stress disorder (PTSD) secondary to sexual abuse, such as hearing voices—often the voice of the perpetrator—panic attacks, eating disorders, nightmares, insomnia, and flashbacks. Studies have concluded that many women who are sexually abused suffer from PTSD (Chu & Dill, 1990; Kendall-Tackett, Williams, & Finkelhor, 1993; Kiser et al., 1988; McCarthy, 1991). But when the women complain about the symptoms of PTSD, they are treated with prescriptions for tranquilizers and psychotropic medications without acknowledgment of the abuse they have suffered or validation of their pain.

Treatment only with medication implies that their emotional problems come from inside of their heads and devalues their sense of victimization, as well as the pain that results from abuse. These drugs thus control a population of women in great need, quieting their complaints without addressing their symptoms. Hence, sexual abuse, which recreates a profound sense of uncontrollability, acts as a violent stressor on the lives of women in prison, denying women power over their sexuality as well as all the other parts of their lives. This humiliation itself compounds the stress of confinement (Laundenslager, Ryan, Drugan, Hyson, & Maier, 1983; Waites, 1993).

In order to cope with the symptoms of their trauma, some survivors of sexual assault become addicted to drugs as a strategy for survival. But, in prison, women do not have access to these drugs, and those who used on the outside face profound waves of depression and anxiety related to their past traumas (Ader & Cohen, 1982; Plotnikoff, 1986; Waites, 1993).

Women who have been battered on the outside carry their pain with them. They suffer from flashbacks when male guards who work in their housing units intimidate them with their size and physical strength. One woman suffered a nervous breakdown after she had been restrained by a male guard because she refused to go to solitary confinement. Women who have been abused and battered are often intimidated by physical force. This intimidation serves as a constant reminder of the helplessness they often experienced while in battering relationships on the outside. And, as on the outside, if women try to fight back, they are labeled "difficult" and punished with isolation. Furthermore, women complain regularly that guards sexually harass and abuse them. Many states insensitively employ male guards in close proximity to female prisoners, and they do not closely supervise their behavior, allowing for the recurrence of violence and abuse.

Children

The children of these invisible women are even more invisible, and their needs are even more ignored. Although most female prisoners are single, separated, widowed, or divorced, most are also mothers. In fact, 80% of women in prison have children. When women go to prison, their children are often left with a grandmother, other relatives, or neighbors who are willing to take care of them. The children become effectively homeless, because, although they have a roof over their heads, they can be moved at any time, and they know this.

The difficulty of making sure that their children are cared for while they are in prison is another great source of stress for the women. Women doing sentences longer than 2 years are at high risk of losing their children, especially if the children are placed in foster care. Imprisonment is considered child neglect, and parental rights can be terminated.

The mental health of women in prison is rarely addressed. Gender stereotypes that inform the decisions made by prison administrators and officials do not help women but instead serve to hinder their access to appropriate therapeutic care. Psychiatrists are often the only mental health care professionals available to women in prison, and they often administer traditional medical diagnoses to depressed women, without reference to the mentally detrimental experiences of incarceration and the separation of a woman from her family, friends, and community. I am convinced that traditional diagnoses such as manic depressive disorder, bipolar personality, and others obscure rather than address the needs of women in prison. The depression that these women experience is often a consequence of their confinement and isolation, and, in many cases, of their withdrawal from dependency on drugs.

A sample of 3,684 inmates in the New York State prison system was surveyed in May 1986 to determine the prevalence of psychiatric and functional disability and service use. It was estimated that 5% had a severe psychiatric disability, and 10% had significant psychiatric disability. The higher the level of disability, the greater the proportion of inmates who had received mental health services in the last 30 days and in the last year. Still, 45% of the severe disability group had no service contacts in the last year. Patterns of use differed significantly by race: A greater proportion of whites received services. The clinical factors associated with receipt of services varied considerably between men and women (Steadman, Holohean, & Dvoskin, 1991).

Each year in the United States, the mothers of 225,000 young children are incarcerated (McGowan & Blumenthal, 1976). On any given day, there are approximately 18,000 women held in federal, state, and local jails and prisons. From 50% to 80% of these women had one or more dependent children living with them, and the women were often the children's primary caretaker at the time of their arrest (Baunach, 1985; Glick & Neto, 1977; McGowan & Blumenthal, 1976; U.S. Comptroller General, 1980). It has been estimated that as many as 80% of those children witness the arrest (Jose, 1985; Stanton, 1980).

Prior to a project I conducted in 1992, there had been no studies on the effects of their mothers' imprisonment on children. With the permission of the mothers and the caretakers, a colleague and I organized such a study, interviewing a group of children whose mothers were incarcerated. We asked them and their caretakers about their feelings about their mother's imprisonment (Jose, 1992). We also gave them standardized tests. We compared these children with others in the same socioeconomic situation who attended the same schools and had many of the same social problems, such as unhealthy living conditions, lack of medical care, poor school performance, and in some cases, mothers who used drugs.

About 75% of children whose mothers were in prison reported symptoms often related to PTSD, such as depression, not doing well in school, sleeping disorders, flashbacks about their mother's arrest or crime, and impaired concentration. As one 12-year-old said, "Since my mother went to prison, things have gone downhill for me." Baunach (1985) found that 70% of the children with mothers in prison were reported as having psychological or emotional problems. "These problems were mainly restlessness, or 'hypertension,' as the mother called it; aggressive behavior; or withdrawal" (p. 31). The psychological impact of separation from a primary caretaker on children of incarcerated mothers also resembles other forms of loss such as divorce or death.

We found that children whose mothers were in prison reported having no emotional support system. For example, when asked who they talked to about problems, 90% of the children answered "nobody."

These children were afraid of causing any problems because they knew that they could always be sent away to another relative's house. They reported symptoms secondary to PTSD, such as lack of sleep and daydreaming at school. They reported remembering every detail of their mother's arrest, as if they were present. They also reported hearing their mother's voice and worrying about their mother's safety.

Some children had not seen their mothers for a year or more until the Children's Visitation Program began. They talked about them as "ghost mothers"—a mother you know you have but you cannot see. Often lack of transportation or the caregiver's belief that the children will get upset when they have to leave stops caregivers from bringing children to visit their mothers in prison. Imprisonment produces tremendous stress for both children and mothers. The mothers worry in prison, and the children worry on the outside.

As with the general population, not all mothers in prison were consistently loving. In fact, some mothers were abusive or neglectful of their children on the outside. This, however, does not mean that the children were not extremely attached to their mothers. In fact, the children we talked to all missed their mothers, even if they remembered negative experiences that they had had when their mothers were at home.

Barbara has spent 11 years in prison. When she talks about her child, her eyes still fill with tears.

> The day that I was arrested is still very vivid in my mind. The day I got picked up to go to jail, I did not want to leave my child with my mother. The thought of my child having to go through all I went through living with my mother. . . It hurt to think of him feeling what I used to feel as a child. Would she beat him up the same way I was? Would he feel lonely and helpless like I felt? All these questions came to my mind. The pain was unbearable. I had no choice. The choices were my mother, where at least I would know what kind of home that was, or someone else that I would not know.

Women in prison are seen as bad mothers. People say, "If they were good mothers, they wouldn't be here." The women in one Midwest prison were required to take parenting classes in order to participate in a special visit with their children. The curriculum was taken from programs aimed at upper-middle class families. The survival techniques that the mothers and their children have to learn are based on an environment of poverty, street violence, and a lack of adequate public and economic resources. The goal for these women is simply to help their children survive. These curriculums are irrelevant to their needs as parents. However, the women take these classes to be able to see their children. If they do not participate, it is held against them as proof that they do not love their children.

Prison is a hard place in which to try to be a parent. Most prisoners have contact with their children only through telephone calls. This gets very expensive for the caretakers, who often have to block the telephone to prevent children from calling their mothers. Writing could be a way to maintain contact, but the prisoners hardly ever receive letters from their children. Writing is hard for the children, and even getting stamps and the mother's address may be difficult for them. The families remain in a constant state of stress produced by the enforced separation of prison life.

Prison and Disease

In addition to the emotional problems that women experience in prison, incarceration creates particular physical health problems. Women are predisposed to develop certain health problems that the experiences of prison confinement encourage. For example, there is a high incidence of hypertension among Black females, with perhaps one in four having high blood pressure. Yet the food in prison is saturated with fats and is likely to exacerbate the already great risk of high blood pressure among the prison population.

The serious overcrowding in prisons leads to the spread of illness, especially tuberculosis and other respiratory diseases. Cramming women into tremendously overcrowded facilities that were not built to provide adequate ventilation puts them at an enormously high risk of infecting each other. One women's prison in Michigan was so overcrowded that 131 women were sleeping in triple bunk beds in the gymnasium, with extremely poor ventilation and light. Such overcrowding, combined with the emotional stress of prison life and the illnesses women bring into the institution, encourages illness to spread rapidly. Prison walls cannot hold these diseases. Women prisoners must be treated as citizens of the world, not simply caged criminals to be forgotten, because their health problems also affect the outside.

HIV and AIDS are special problems in prisons. AZT and other drugs for HIV are expensive and are often not available in prison. HIV and AIDS both present enormous health problems for women, few of which are directly addressed by prison health administrators. HIV has had a devastating impact on low-income Black and Latina women in prison. Moreover, prison health personnel are not trained to look at the different symptoms of HIV-related diseases that women manifest. HIV-positive women are often placed in isolation. When they are allowed to stay in the general prison population, all personnel working with them are advised of their condition, and they are not allowed to work with food. Fear of infection through casual contact is heightened in prison because of the general AIDS-phobic messages that prisoners bring with them from the outside. Thus, in such close quarters, rumors and tensions spread rapidly. Instead of receiving special care and treatment, HIV-positive women are ostracized and denied access to the few resources available to women in prison. For example, inmates in one prison petitioned the administration to move a prisoner who was HIV-positive into solitary confinement, where she would have no access to any emotional resources. Officers who moved her to another unit wore gloves and masks, feeding the misconception that HIV can be spread through casual contact.

Conclusions

The need to design programs that are specific to Latina and African American women prisoners cannot be debated any longer. Culturally sensitive programs need to address the therapeutic and physical needs of women, respecting the fact that many inmates had been traumatized by sexual violence on the outside.

Women in prison suffer from lack of health care appropriate to their gender and social conditions. Women prisoners' bodies and minds are at the mercy of the institution that holds them and controls their access to medical care. Prison is a reflection of society—a magnification of the sexism, racism, and classism perpetuated on our most oppressed sisters and their children. Women in prison and their health must be taken as an important issue in the women's and health rights movements. To forget women in prison would not only contribute to the oppression that they suffer in society but would also deny the central role that they play in the dynamics of this country.

Prisons and prisoners are as integral to the American imagination as the myth of their invisibility. As we continue to pretend that women in prison are marginal and unimportant, we perpetuate a lie that upholds the distinctions between the "good" and the "bad" in our society, and we lend implicit support to a system that denies health care and civil rights to anyone who is marginalized. We end up reinforcing the disenfranchisement of women of color, of poor women, and of women who have been caught in a system that denies them their personhood. Thus, as we forget the injustices that women in prison face, we are reproducing the frustration and humiliation that they face in prison. We are not listening to their needs or thinking about how race contributes to their oppression. Instead, we are contributing to their disempowerment at the hands of a system that claims it has the resources only to control their bodies, not to maintain their health. Thus, women in prison are not bad, they are not criminal, they are not symbolic. They are women whose civil rights and access to health care are denied on the inside, as they were on the outside. Race and socioeconomic class denied these women access to adequate health care before they walked through the prison gates and continue to work to their disadvantage on the inside. They are women who are manipulated by a rigid and lumbering bureaucracy. Ultimately, if we forget the health needs of Latinas and other women in prison, our fight for justice for all women and all people is rendered incomplete and unjust.

Women are often released from prison with poor health and undiagnosed diseases. Although conventional wisdom would suggest that pinching pennies on health care will save in overall prison costs, experience has shown that a dollar of public money spent on prevention and diagnosis will save hundreds of dollars on medical intervention and emergency services. Most prison inmates are released into economically deprived communities where they find themselves disadvantaged even in comparison to other residents. Women who are released from prison often find themselves alienated from the communities that they left behind, and without other kinds of resources like jobs or health care. Health is difficult to maintain in substandard housing, and health care is difficult to come by, especially preventive care.

The health care of these women should be managed by the criminal justice system itself. Governmental agencies should take care of women who have recently been released from jail by offering them emotional support and government-sponsored health service to take care of them. Women in prison should have access to health care on the outside as well. Also, problems of alcohol and drug abuse must be addressed from the women's own perspective, through programs in the prison. But these programs need to be tied to the community so that there is some link between women's experiences and support in and outside of prison.

Ultimately, health care reforms must include women in prison and their children. Without this form of support, women in the criminal justice system and their children are condemned to poor nutrition, poor health, and poverty due to these problems. We must stop the cycle of poor health for women in prison.

References

Ader, R., & Cohen, N. (1982). Behaviorally conditioned immunosuppression and murine systemic lupus erythematosis. *Science, 215*, 1534-1536.

Baunach, P. J. (1985). *Mothers in prison*. New Brunswick, NJ: Transaction Books.

Chu, J. A., & Dill, D. L. (1990). Dissociative symptoms in relation to childhood physical and sexual abuse. *American Journal of Psychiatry, 147*, 887-892.

Deming, B. (1966). *Prison notes*. New York: Grossman.

Foucault, M. (1979). *Discipline and punish: The birth of the prison*. New York: Random House.

Glaser, J. B., Greifinger, R. B. (1993). Correctional health care: A public health opportunity. *Annals of Internal Medicine, 118*(2), 139-145.

Glick, R., & Neto, V. V. (1977). *National study of women's correctional programs*. Washington, DC: National Institute of Law Enforcement and Criminal Justice.

Jose, C. (1985). *Women doing life sentences: A phenomenological study*. Unpublished dissertation, University of Michigan, Ann Arbor.

Jose, C. (1992). *Children of incarcerated mothers: The voiceless children*. Unpublished manuscript.

Kendall-Tackett, K. A., Williams, L. M., & Finkelhor, D. (1993). The impact of sexual abuse on children: A review and synthesis of recent empirical studies. *Psychology Bulletin, 113,* 164-180.

Kiser, L. J., Ackerman, B. J., Brown, E., Edwards, N. B., McColgan, E., Pugh, R., & Pruitt, D. B. (1988). Post-traumatic stress disorder in children: A reaction to purported sexual abuse. *Journal of the American Academy of Child and Adolescent Psychiatry, 27,* 645-649.

Laudenslager, M. L., Ryan, S. M., Drugan, R. C., Hyson, R. L., & Maier, S. F. (1983). Coping and immunosuppression: Inescapable but not escapable shock suppresses lymphocyte proliferation. *Science, 221,* 568-570.

McCarthy J. B. (1991). Survivors of physical and sexual abuse. *American Journal of Orthopsychiatry, 61,* 475-477.

McGaha, G. S. (1986). Correctional health care: Beyond the barriers. *Journal of Offender Counseling, Services and Rehabilitation, 10.*

McGowan, B. G., & Blumenthal, K. L. (1978). *Why punish the children? A study of children of women in prison.* Trenton: New Jersey Council of Delinquency.

Michigan Women's Commission. (1987). *Women in Michigan: Statistical portrait of women in the state of Michigan.* Ann Arbor: Institute for Social Research, University of Michigan.

Plotnikoff, N. P. (1986). *Enkephalins and endorphins: Stress and the immune system.* New York: Plenum.

Rafter, N. H. (1985). *Partial justice: Women in state prisons, 1800-1935.* Boston: Northeastern University Press.

Stanton, A. M. (1980). *When mothers go to jail.* Lexington, MA: Lexington Books.

Steadman, H. J., Holohean, E. J., Jr., & Dvoskin, J. (1991). Estimating mental health needs and service utilization among prison inmates. *Bulletin of American Academic Psychiatry and Law, 19*(3), 297-307.

U. S. Comptroller General. (1980). *Women in prison: Inequitable treatment requires action.* Washington, DC: General Accounting Office.

U.S. Office of the Surgeon General. (1993). *One voice, one vision: Recommendations to the Surgeon General to improve Hispanic/Latino health.* Washington, DC: Author.

Waites, E. A. (1993). *Trauma and survival: Post-traumatic and dissociative disorders in women.* New York: Norton.

11 The Impact of Homelessness Among Women of Color

DIANE L. ADAMS

MARGARET S. MASON

A serious health crisis steadily plagues us and can no longer be ignored—the condition of homelessness. Although we are faced with daily demonstrations of this condition, a consistent definition of homelessness eludes us. Many have tried to define what constitutes a homeless person. A scientific study designed to count the homeless population of Chicago defined homelessness as "a manifestation of extreme poverty among persons *without families* in housing markets with declining stocks of inexpensive dwelling units suitable for single persons" (Rossi, Wright, Fisher, & Willis, 1987, p. 1336).

According to the Stewart B. McKinney Homeless Assistance Act of 1987, a homeless person is (a) an individual who lacks a fixed, regular, and adequate nighttime residence; or (b) an individual who has a primary night-time residency that is one of the following:

1. a supervised publicly or privately operated shelter designed to provide temporary living accommodations (including welfare hotels, congregate shelters, and transitional housing for the mentally ill);

2. an institution that provides a temporary residence for individuals intended to be institutionalized; or

3. a public or private place not designated for, or ordinarily used as, regular sleeping accommodations for human beings.

This term does not include any individual imprisoned or otherwise detained under an Act of Congress or a state law (U.S. Department of Housing and Urban Development, 1994, p. 22).

The National Governors Association defined a homeless person as "an undomiciled person who is unable to secure permanent and stable housing without special assistance" (Kennedy et al., 1990, p. 86). The U.S. General Accounting Office defined homeless individuals as those who lack resources and community ties necessary to provide for their own adequate shelter (Kennedy et al., 1990).

All of these definitions attempt to describe the homeless population, yet when research efforts are undertaken, varying interpretations are used to structure sampling and counting methodologies. This results in underreporting of the number of people in need.

Meanwhile, the number of homeless families continues to grow at an ever-increasing rate, due primarily to problems related to health and socioeconomic factors. Approximately 40% of the homeless population is made up of family members with children, 75% of whom are women with children.

Although there are various service alternatives in place to address the needs of the homeless, such as shelter based-clinics, school-based clinics, mobile health units, and emergency rooms, a transitional system of care for this vulnerable population is missing. Consequently, a number of questions relevant to this epidemic go unanswered:

Who are the homeless?

When did they become homeless?

Why did they become homeless?

Where are they geographically located?

What is being done to address their health care needs?

How can we improve their access to appropriate and culturally sensitive quality health care?

Chapters 12, 13, and 14 raise issues related to the health of women and children of color who are homeless. Both mental health concerns and economic factors that contribute to their homeless condition will be discussed.

References

Kennedy, J. T., Petrone, J., Deisher, R. W., Emerson, J., Heslop, P., Bastible, D., & Arkovitz, M. (1990). Health care for familyless, runaway street kids. In P. W. Breckner, L. K. Scharer, B. A. Conanan, M. Savarese, & B. C. Scanlan (Eds.), *Under the safety net: The health and social welfare of the homeless in the United States* (pp. 82-117). New York: Norton.

Rossi, P. H., Wright, J. D., Fisher, G. A., & Willis, G. (1987). The urban homeless: Estimating composition and size. *Science, 234*(4794), 1336-1341.

U.S. Department of Housing & Urban Development. (1994). *Priority: Home! The federal plan to break the cycle of homelessness* (Publication No. HUD-1454-CPD). Washington, DC: Author.

12 The Growth of Homelessness in America

Health Concerns

SHANELL SEMIEN

SHANNON SEMIEN

Homelessness in the United States today is a far different issue from the homelessness of several decades ago. It is a serious issue with profound health implications. Within the span of two decades, homelessness has become one of this country's major social and health challenges. It has been transformed from a minor urban condition, experienced predominantly by males and observed in skid row neighborhoods, to a condition experienced by some 8.5 million Americans in the period between 1985 and 1990 (Rosenbeck, 1994). Furthermore, an ever-increasing percentage of this growing number of homeless individuals are women, women with children, and homeless families.

The present problem of homelessness first came to public awareness during the 1980s, when the deep recession from 1982 to 1983

NOTE: This chapter is the maiden voyage for two college seniors soon to enter the professional world, whom the editor felt deserved an opportunity to be published. Advisers to the students were Diane L. Adams and Margaret S. Mason.

brought what was thought to be a temporary rise in unemployment and homelessness. Because the rise in unemployment was expected to be short-lived, many people also expected homelessness to be short-lived, a crisis that would go away when business and times improved. This, however, was not the case. During the late 1980s, when the country experienced a period of sustained growth that was the longest in the postwar years, homelessness did not disappear, nor did its growth abate. Rather, the face of the homeless population underwent a complete metamorphosis—a drastic change in age and gender.

The age of homeless persons sharply declined: In the 1950s and 1960s, the homeless were usually males in their mid-50s; in the 1980s, the homeless were in their mid-30s, and homeless single women, women with children, and homeless families were more in evidence. Yet the condition of homelessness continued to be seen as a peripheral issue related to marginal populations in large urban centers.

Homelessness was widely viewed as a temporary problem, confined to the forgotten fringes of society and not affecting the societal core. The homeless were seen as being to blame for their condition. They were stigmatized as suffering from personal deficits and having dramatic personal problems that caused their homelessness. Many studies highlighted the facts that homeless people were mentally ill and often suffered from substance abuse disorders and severe social isolation and that many were members of racial minority groups. The homeless were portrayed as rebels and involuntary exiles who could but would not participate in the social mainstream (Marin, 1987).

President Ronald Reagan suggested that the homeless were deviants who chose their homeless lifestyles voluntarily; this attitude further distorted the image of the homeless. He reassured the American public that many jobs were available, as indicated by the want ads in the typical Sunday paper, for those motivated homeless workers who would make the effort required to apply (Rosenbeck, 1994). Meanwhile, the problem of homelessness continued to grow exponentially as it progressed forward to present-day proportions.

The study of Link and his colleagues (1994) painted a different picture of homelessness. They saw homelessness as a national phenomenon of broad scope. Based upon a nationwide telephone survey of representative U.S. households, Link et al. estimated that 13.5 million adults had experienced homelessness, 5.7 million of them between 1985 and 1990. The authors found the condition of homelessness to be no greater among men than women, among Blacks than Whites, or among urban than rural populations.

This national study, unlike others, suggested not an aberrant phenomenon affecting only the down and out in urban centers, but a major change in our society as a whole, accompanied by the deindustrialization of the economy (Rosenbeck, 1994). The results of deindustrialization were evident in several areas. Those who lack both education and skills now find that employment opportunities have drastically declined (Mishel & Frankel, 1993). African American neighborhoods, once diverse, thriving settings, are now characterized by concentrated poverty (Massey & Denton, 1993). Unemployment is higher in some rural areas than in some urban areas (Bluestone & Harrison, 1982). Small farmers have been displaced from their land (Link et al., 1994).

In another development of the 1980s, Mishel and Frankel (1993) found that those at the lower end of the socioeconomic scale experienced a 13% decline in income, while those at the higher end experienced an 8% increase. This observation is substantiated by the number of low-income people across the country who fall below the poverty level and are unable to make ends meet, although they work every day. These include women with children and families who are homeless. The U.S. Bureau of the Census (1992b) bears this out. In 1990, poverty affected 31.9% of all Blacks and 35.5% of all Black women. Single-parent, female-headed households constituted 44% of all Black households, and their poverty was greater than that of the Black population as a whole. About 48% of Black female-headed families had income below the poverty level, and 75% of the 2 million Black families in poverty in 1990 were maintained by women without a husband present (U.S. Bureau of the Census, 1992a).

The study by Link et al. (1994) establishes clearly that the magnitude of the problem of homelessness is greater than we may have been led to believe. No longer can homelessness be defined as simply residence on skid row. The definition of homelessness has changed. The current definition reflects primarily those completely without shelter or those living in homeless shelters who would otherwise be without a place to sleep. It includes not only a younger population but also a population of homeless women and their families.

Pursuant to this new definition of homelessness, this chapter focuses on the relationship of low educational achievement and poverty to health, the relationship of the living environment of the homeless to health, health problems of the homeless, access to health care among the homeless, and health promotion and disease prevention among the homeless.

Lack of Education, Poverty, and Health

The condition of homelessness is rarely an isolated event but may be viewed as the culmination of a process. Homelessness for most individuals is experienced at the end of a series of conditions, all of which impinge on health. Lack of education, illiteracy, very low educational achievement, and lack of skill development can all function as springboards to poverty.

People lacking in educational achievement or skill development suffer long-term unemployment or frequent episodes of unemployment. They have very low earning potential and are limited in their ability to hold a job above the minimum-wage level. They often work at very dangerous jobs. Although such people may work every day, they find themselves below the poverty level, constantly struggling to make ends meet—without success. They find the earnings from a minimum-wage job insufficient to support the typical minimal expenses of food, shelter, and utilities.

The impact of this condition is inadequate housing, malnutrition, and little or no health insurance, resulting in little or no preventive health care. The stresses of constant struggle for African Americans translate into the highest rate of depression of any ethnic group (Liu & Yu, 1985), low self-esteem, and high levels of anxiety.

Women find themselves homeless when they are evicted, separated from their mates because of abuse to themselves or to their children, or separated from their children because of domestic difficulties, which can result in their losing Aid to Families With Dependent Children (AFDC) support. Sudden loss of employment or a sudden, uninsured, costly illness may render an entire family homeless.

Lack of education may also be a factor in the condition of homelessness for elderly women. Homelessness among the elderly varies from other populations in that it is the culmination of a series of events marked by a gradual loss of social support and increasing disaffiliation. Elderly women who are evicted from their homes may then experience mental illness, relationship cutoffs, death of the mate or caregiver, relocation, and loss of income (Sullivan, 1991). The homeless elderly fall into two categories. They may be part of a smaller group of totally unsheltered or so-called street people who lack a fixed nighttime address, or they may be part of a group of marginally housed elderly whose living arrangements are unstable and place them in imminent danger of becoming homeless. Other factors that may be related to homelessness among the elderly are alcoholism, physical illness, and lack of support systems (Weiss, 1992).

Living Environments of
the Homeless—Health Implications

Both the existence of and the number of homeless people in this country are important issues and challenges to public health. This problem did not develop overnight, nor will it disappear overnight. Homelessness poses severe challenges for the control of infectious diseases and puts homeless people at risk of physical and mental health problems.

Locating people once they have become homeless is a daunting task in itself. The homeless population consists of a diverse group of individuals who may be found in many different and unexpected places. The homeless are found not only in shelters but in boxcars, on the roofs of tenements, in campgrounds, under bridges and freeway overpasses, and in garages, abandoned buildings, bus terminals, airports, cars, vans, and buses. Families living in transitional housing, one step removed from the condition of homelessness, are often technically considered homeless. Some homeless people deliberately hide the fact that they are homeless when being interviewed, out of embarrassment. Other people experience short or intermittent episodes of homelessness. Still others move in with relatives and friends, creating overcrowded living and sleeping conditions that quicken the spread of communicable diseases. All these living environments put the homeless at tremendous risk for various mental and physical health problems and disorders.

Illness and Health Disorders of the Homeless

For the homeless population, access to health care is problematic and limited. According to Usatine, Gelberg, Smith, and Lesser (1994), homeless people often seek health care too late or not at all, and they may fear visiting hospital emergency facilities because of previous bad experiences with the health care system. They are afraid of being turned away because of lack of money or insurance, and they may even lack the transportation to get to places where health services are offered. The homeless are often embarrassed to present themselves to caregivers in the disheveled and often unclean state resulting from their homeless condition.

Usatine et al. (1994) provide a detailed look at the leading health problems in homeless adults. The problems discussed include the following:

Upper respiratory infections: tuberculosis, pneumococcal pneumonia and diphtheria

Skin ailments: impetigo, eczema, a fungal infection called *tinea pedis* (an infection of the toes), transmission of scabies and lice

Chronic gastrointestinal disorder: diarrhea

Genitourinary problems: urinary tract infection

Peripheral vascular problems: cellulitis and leg ulcers

Dental disorders: caries, gingivitis, abscesses

Neurological disorders: alcoholism and drug abuse

Weather-related conditions: hypothermia, heat stroke, and sunburns

Traumatic injuries resulting from crime-related behavior: lacerations, abrasions, rape, and sometime death

Malnutrition is very common among the homeless and may be the result of limited access to food, poor quality of food, alcoholism, drug abuse, or mental illness, including personality and anxiety disorders, acute depressive disorders, and co-morbidity (mental disorder and substance abuse). The inability to follow a specific diet results in aggravated diabetes, hypertension, or hyperlipidemia. Other health-related risk factors include sexually transmitted diseases (STDs) and human immunodeficiency virus/acquired immune deficiency syndrome (HIV/AIDS).

Homeless women with children are less likely to be emotionally unstable and less likely to be substance abusers than homeless women without children. Homeless families are less likely to suffer problems associated with drug and alcohol abuse. Their homelessness is more likely to be associated with sudden loss of employment or an uninsured health emergency.

Access to Health Care Among the Homeless

In general, homeless women do not use public health care clinics for primary health care. Some factors that contribute to homeless women's nonuse of primary care services are inconvenient clinic hours, cost, and lack of transportation. Even when some of these factors are eliminated, homeless women may still hesitate to seek health care. Unfriendly and rude health care providers create unpleasant experiences and barriers to health care.

Health care providers may think that homeless people are to blame for their condition or that the poor are not engaging in health promotion and health prevention activities or being compliant with their medical regimens. Health care providers who are insensitive, judgmental, sexist, rude, or hostile create barriers for the poor and the homeless (Ugarriza & Fallon, 1994). These attitudes and behaviors discourage the homeless from seeking much needed health care.

Health Promotion and Disease
Prevention Among the Homeless

Health promotion and disease prevention are of great importance to homeless patients. There is a significant need for adequate low-cost community-based health organizations to strengthen community contact/connection with health caregivers. It is likely that the home-less would seek care in a familiar community setting. Effective com-munity-based organizations would do well to plan and implement strategies that encourage the use of available health services (Voelker, 1994). Services to develop health care promotion and intervention programs should be culturally sensitive. The services should avoid creating unreasonable fears or promoting distrust based on race, ethnicity, religion, social class, gender, or sexual orientation. More-over, the services should promote confidence in the health care system and a feeling of acceptance and well-being. In addition, programs should be evaluated for their attention to ethical values, as well as for their effectiveness.

Professional associations of health care providers can take on the responsibility for educating members about the needs of poor and homeless women. Such activities as seminars, continuing education, community outreach programs, charitable and research grants, and awards focused on intervention strategies for poor women would be effective in reducing barriers to care. Professional care providers could work to persuade curriculum developers in their alma mater graduate schools to include courses that focus on the health problems, both physical and emotional, common to homeless women. Health care professionals themselves can motivate poor and homeless women to seek care by providing encouragement, education, and a caring attitude (Ugarriza & Fallon, 1994).

Conclusion

There is a paucity of data specifically targeting homelessness among women of color. What is known is that illiteracy/low educa-tion, lack of skill development, unemployment/sporadic employ-ment, minimum wage work, and poverty are antecedents to home-lessness. Women of color are disproportionately represented among those who experience these antecedents; we can therefore expect them to be significantly represented among homeless women, home-less women with children, and women with homeless families.

References

Bluestone, B., & Harrison B. (1982). *The deindustrialization of America: Plant closings, community abandonment, and the dismantling of basic industry*. New York: Basic Books.

Link, B. G., Susser, E., Stueve, A., Phelan, J., Moore, R. E., & Struening, E. (1994). Lifetime and five-year prevalence of homelessness in the United States. *American Journal of Public Health, 84*, 1907-1912.

Liu, W. T., & Yu, E. S. H. (1985). Ethnicity, mental health, and the urban delivery system. In L. Maldonado & J. Moore (Eds.), *Urban ethnicity in the United States* (pp. 211-247). Beverly Hills, CA: Sage.

Marin, P. (1987, January). Helping and hating the homeless. *Harper's*, pp. 39-49.

Massey, D. A., & Denton, N. A. (1993). *American apartheid: Segregation and the making of the underclass*. Cambridge, MA: Harvard University Press.

Mishel, L., & Frankel, D. M. (1993). *The state of working America: 1992-1993*. New York: M. E. Sharpe.

Rosenbeck, R. (1994). Editorials and annotations. *American Journal of Public Health, 84*, 1885-1886.

Sullivan, M. A. (1991). Homeless older women in context: Alienation, cutoff, and reconnection. *Journal of Women and Aging, 3*, 3-24.

Ugarriza, D. N., & Fallon, T. (1994). Nurses' attitudes toward homeless women: A barrier to change. *Nursing Outlook, 42*, 26-29.

Usatine, R. P., Gelberg, G., Smith, M. H., & Lesser, J. (1994). Health care for the homeless: A family medicine perspective. *American Family Physician, 49*, 139-146.

U.S. Bureau of the Census. (1992a). *The Black population in the United States: March 1991* (Current population reports, Series P-20, No.464). Washington, DC: Government Printing Office.

U.S. Bureau of the Census. (1992b). *Statistical abstract of the United States* (112th ed.). Washington, DC: Government Printing Office.

Voelker, R. (1994). Community-based health care for the homeless. *Journal of the American Medical Association, 271* (19), 1496.

Weiss, L. M. (1992). *There's no place like . . . no place: Confronting the problems of the aging, homeless, and marginally housed*. Washington, DC: American Association of Retired Persons.

13 Mental Health Problems of Women of Color Who Are Homeless

PHYLLIS OLD DOG CROSS

Concern about the homeless women and children of America and awareness of their plight are growing. A survey by the Department of Housing and Urban Development noted in 1988 that 40% of the homeless population is made up of families with children; of this group, 75% are women with children (Homeless Information Exchange, 1993). Fewer data are available concerning women of color who are homeless. One study of the homeless in New York City found that, of all the men interviewed, 76% were African American; of all the women interviewed, 74% were African American; and of the total, 75.6% were African American (Herman, Struening, & Barrow, 1994). In a paper presented at the 122nd Annual Conference of the American Public Health Association, Marion E. Primas (1994) said that 51% of the homeless are African American, while Hispanics, Asians, and Native Americans together make up 14%. No data were available from rural areas and Indian reservations.

Mental health, or lack of it, is an important part of the problems of homeless women of color (Herman et al., 1994). The leading cause of homelessness is domestic violence (Homeless Information Exchange,

1994). Other data show that between 25% and 50% of homeless women are trying to escape abusive partners (Bussiere, Freedman, Menning, Mihaly, & Morales, 1991). A common occurrence in domestic violence is that the woman must leave the home to save herself from further abuse. She has the choice of life without resources or returning to a dangerous situation.

The psychological profile of an abused woman reveals that she has lowered self-esteem and feelings of hopelessness, shame, and self-blame. She is usually chronically depressed as a result of years of physical and emotional abuse. Her coping skills and ability to deal with life's problems have been greatly diminished (Homeless Information Exchange, 1994).

Mental Illness. Mental illness is mentioned frequently as an issue that needs to be addressed. A study that compared homeless women with children to housed mothers with children found the homeless were more frequently abused, had more problems with alcohol, and had more serious psychiatric problems (Bassuk & Rosenburg, 1988). Another study that assessed self-reported needs of homeless people found that mental health and substance abuse ranked high as problems (Herman et al., 1994).

Racism. Several authors have addressed the issue of racism as experienced by women of color (Anzaldua, 1990). Racism affects not only the internal psyche but also the provision of services. Women of color receive less health care than white women do (Watson, 1994). The literature about women of color documents how they are being treated (Moraga & Anzaldua, 1981) and gives voice to the inner rage they feel as a result of years of exposure to racism.

Anxiety. Anxiety usually accompanies depression or stress situations, according to the *Diagnostic and Statistical Manual of Mental Disorders* (American Psychiatric Association, 1987, p. 251). Women experiencing all or some of the many emotional stressors of homelessness can display severe anxiety. Symptoms of fear, restlessness, agitation, crying, weight loss, lack of sleep, and indecisiveness are present. Anxiety can be so severe that the person becomes dysfunctional. The victim may experience anxiety attacks so severe that she may fear she is dying. Anxiety can be manifested in many physical symptoms, headaches, stomach problems, and unexplained pain. Untreated or ignored anxiety can become chronic, and many self-medicate to find relief. The mental health needs of homeless women of color have been noted before. Treatment of anxiety, as well as its causes, is a basic need for these women (Old Dog Cross, 1985).

Depression. Depression is a common illness that affects a large number of people, homeless or not. In the general population, the range for females is from 9% to 26%, and for males 5% to 12% (*DSM-III-R*, 1987, p. 229). Depression affects women twice as much as men (*DSM-III-R*, 1987, p. 229). It is a syndrome usually related to a loss or series of losses, such as death of a loved one, loss of possessions, and financial problems.

Depression is manifested in the sufferer by feelings of hopelessness, anxiety, loss of self-esteem, guilt, shame, sleeplessness, feelings of worthlessness, and loss of appetite. The emotional and physical pain connected to depression is sometimes so acute that the depressed person may choose to end it by suicide (*DSM-III-R*, 1987, p. 228).

Homeless women of color have already suffered severe emotional stress and loss. Their coping skills are weak. Among them are the abused and the elderly, who may be both solitary and homeless. Because depression often results from these situations, it could be suggested that many women of color need attention by trained mental health personnel for evaluation and, if necessary, treatment.

Posttraumatic Stress Disorder. Posttraumatic stress disorder (PTSD), once only diagnosed in soldiers recovering from combat in war, now is recognized to occur in people who have experienced emotional or physical trauma. This trauma may include incidents of rape, battering, and sexual trauma. Flashbacks are a frequent symptom of PTSD; victims complain of reliving the traumatic incident, which triggers the same reactions the original event caused. Victims experience fear and confusion. They may become chronically depressed and anxious and experience sleep deprivation, hopelessness, shame, and for some, thoughts of self-destruction. PTSD can also occur after other acts of violence and after disasters such as floods (*DSM-III-R*, 1987, p. 247).

Women of color who experience PTSD should be given special attention to help them understand the causes of their symptoms.

Suicide. People who are under severe emotional stress and suffering from a variety of problems may turn to thoughts of suicide as the possible solution. Some actually do choose self-destruction. For instance, the suicide rate for Native Americans is several times that of the general population (May, 1987). Homeless people suffer from depression, anxiety, mental illness, and drug abuse. These are all problems that might lead homeless women of color to consider suicide as a solution to their problems. The inner feelings of abandonment, rejection, shame, loneliness, and hopelessness cause the sufferer to seek relief from the pain. A woman who is mentally ill might hear voices telling her to kill herself. A drug abuser or alcoholic in the pain of withdrawal might "give up" and seek out death. Suicide attempts are referred to as a cry for help. They certainly are a signal that a human being is in pain (May, 1987).

To manage potentially suicidal people or the people with suicidal intent, the caretaker must take them seriously. It is important not to ridicule them or to agitate them. Every effort must be made to get homeless women of color to an expert in mental health care. If there is a language barrier or cultural differences, this also must be taken into account (DeBruyn, Hymbaugh, & Valdez, 1988). It is recommended that women of color have access to adequate mental health care and emergency mental health care to prevent suicide.

Chronic Mental Illness. Chronic mental illness (CMI) has been cited over and over as one of the major problems in dealing with the homeless (Bassuk & Rosenburg, 1988; Liebow, 1993; Primas, 1994). CMI is a rather general term lumping together various serious mental disorders, including schizophrenia, bipolar disorder, personality disorder, and psychotic depression. It is often seen combined with substance abuse problems; then it is called a dual-diagnosis disorder, which will be discussed separately. At times, an organic brain disorder may also be present (*DSM-III-R*, 1987, p. 119).

Much has been published regarding the deinstitutionalization of CMI patients in the 1960s and 1970s (Sullivan, 1992). The movement to return patients to their home communities had several goals: to stop warehousing patients, to move patients closer to their home communities, to help patients enjoy a better quality of life (Reissman, Cohen, & Pearl, 1964). The movement was part of the Community Mental Health Centers Act of 1963 (PL 88-164). Staff were to establish after-care programs, one of the six essential services they were to provide. Patients who were in large state mental hospitals for many years were sent home for care. But for many reasons, mentally ill people drifted into the group known as "street people" or homeless. What started as a humane movement to free chronic patients from institutions ended with these people homeless on the streets, victims of their disease (Government Accounting Office, 1977; Gulati, 1992).

Schizophrenia. Many homeless people suffer from schizophrenia, a severe mental disorder that is related to a brain disorder of unknown cause. It is characterized by bizarre behavior, hallucinations of all kinds, intense paranoia, fear, and suspiciousness. Often intricate patterns of paranoid thinking cause sufferers to imagine people are plotting to harm them. The classic "bag lady" who is disheveled, yelling strange words, and pushing a large cart of "stuff" is usually a victim of this severe mental illness (*DSM-III-R*, 1987, p. 225).

Bipolar Disorder. Bipolar disorder is a disease of the brain, formerly known as manic depressive illness. It is characterized by mood swings and is considered a severe mental disorder (*DSM-III-R*, 1987, p. 225). In the manic phase, a woman might display exhibitionistic behavior and express grandiose ideas, plans, and schemes. She may act out sexually or spend money lavishly. The woman in the full manic stage is difficult to manage and control; she may become paranoid and delusional, and she may be dangerous. The woman with bipolar disorder frequently uses drugs or alcohol to self-medicate. It is recommended that women of color who have this disorder be given access to treatment. They will need the services of a psychiatrist, laboratory, and pharmacy. This disorder can be treated and managed effectively.

Psychiatric Medication. Mention should be made here that many mentally ill women who are homeless can be treated successfully with medication. Physicians prescribe various psychiatric drugs to help control symptoms and relieve the anxiety of mental illness. Some medications lessen or eradicate the paranoia and hallucinations of schizophrenia and psychotic depression. The medication must be monitored by a responsible person. Side effects of various medications can be serious and should be observed closely. One unfortunate side effect is *tardive dyskinesia*, which causes involuntary facial movements. Proper care for women of color who are homeless means good mental health follow-up and access to mental health care. There must also be access to medication and provision of supervision (Koegel, 1987).

Organic Brain Syndrome. Organic brain syndrome (OBS) is a disorder of the brain caused by various kinds of trauma, including alcoholism, inhalants, toxic substance, malnutrition, some physical illnesses, and violent head injuries. Symptoms can include mild to severe memory loss, disorientation, seizures, and physical disability. These symptoms sometimes are bizarre enough to cause the victim to be ostracized or abused by others. Often the person is labeled crazy (*DSM-III-R*, 1987, p. 119). OBS can sometimes be treated with medication, although it may also be irreversible. The best treatment requires a compassionate, humane approach.

Substance Abuse. Abuse of substances, including alcohol, inhalants, and other drugs, is common among the homeless. In fact, the stereotype of the "street bum" is the chronic alcoholic. Women of color who are homeless are reported to have a problem with substance abuse (Primas, 1994). Mind-altering substances may temporarily relieve the stress of the present; the symptoms of anxiety, depression, and PTSD are lessened.

Continued use of these substances can result in addiction, with all its problems. Continued use of alcohol can result in chronic symptoms of alcoholism and even death. Use of inhalants can result in severe OBS. Use of hard drugs such as heroin, speed, and others can also result in severe mental and physical problems. Use of intravenous needles can expose homeless women to AIDS.

Dual Diagnosis. A person who is chronically mentally ill and also uses chemical substances is referred to as a dual diagnosis client (Primas,

1994). A large number of mentally ill homeless people are considered to have dual diagnosis problems, and they pose unique problems for treatment facilities. Many psychiatric programs are unable to deal with the alcoholic patient and are not equipped to deal with detoxification. Alcohol treatment facilities cannot cope with the chronic psychiatric woman patient. There is now agreement that both problems should be treated simultaneously, but programs that can do so are rare.

Fetal Alcohol Syndrome and Fetal Alcohol Effect. Fetal alcohol syndrome (FAS) and fetal alcohol effect (FAE) are two disorders caused by the mother's drinking of alcohol during pregnancy (May, Hymbaugh, Aase, & Samet, 1985). This particular mental health problem among women of color is mentioned here because it is now being recognized both as a problem for pregnant women of color and also for those suffering from FAS and FAE (Health Care for Homeless Information Center, 1992).

Focus has been placed on Native American women and their drinking patterns, but FAS and FAE are found in and create problems among all races. Because of their gender, women respond differently than men to alcohol; for instance, female alcoholics are eight times more likely to commit suicide than non-alcoholic women. Also, Native American women have the highest rates of death from cirrhosis (Indian Health Service, 1985). Special attention must focus on women of color to deal with prevention of FAS and FAE. Studies and research efforts must be directed to this problem.

Psychosocial Aspects of Aging: Women of Color. The process of aging causes difficulties, both physical and psychosocial, even for a person who is living a somewhat normal life. A person who feels the effects of the aging process along with all the trials of being homeless can experience severe distress (Birch, 1985). Aging women are prone to falls and experience a lack of strength and loss of vigor that may be compounded by exposure and poor nutrition. They may be prone to osteoarthritis or osteoporosis. Poor vision and loss of hearing may also contribute to confusion and falls.

Aging women may experience some memory loss, especially involving recent recall. Although for some the loss is slight, others find the loss so severe that they become confused and disoriented. The confusion may be due to excessive alcohol or drug abuse. Malnutrition can also cause these organic brain symptoms. The severest problem of all is Alzheimer's syndrome, a condition that is considered to be genetic. It is progressive and ends in total confusion, combativeness, and eventually death.

In addition to the physical aspects of aging, homeless women often experience depression that ranges from mild to severe. The various overwhelming losses they experience, such as death of loved ones, illness, loss of a home, and loss of physical health, may lead to a grief reaction and depression that includes feelings of hopelessness, shame, loss of self-esteem, and loneliness. Aging homeless women of color may also be mentally ill, a problem discussed in other parts of this chapter. OBS may cause bizarre behavior and a condition called dementia can occur.

Access to Mental Health Services

Accessing services for mental health problems in the homeless population is itself problematic. Access includes elements of finance, culture, geography, and eligibility. Even if homeless women of color choose to seek help, the barriers can be almost insurmountable for many (Lamb, 1984). First of all, homeless women of color must locate a public mental health clinic, determine if they are eligible and meet guidelines, and then keep the appointment, arrange transportation, and arrange for child care, if necessary. They may have to go through an intake process and be assigned to a specific therapist for return visits. Medication may be prescribed, and the women must find a way to purchase it. Finally, if hospitalization or special tests are required, another barrier must be faced (Kunitz, Levy, & Harwood, 1981).

Problems encountered at the place providing mental health services may include a language barrier. Some Native Americans communicate only in their tribal language; some Asian groups also encounter problems. Cultural beliefs and practices can also present barriers. Women of color might be going to a medicine man, *cuandero*, or native healer, and using native medicines; the therapist might reject the client's beliefs as witchcraft or voodoo (Carnicorm, 1982). Also, the mental health care provider might be of the predominant culture and not be trusted by women of color. They may have experienced various insults from the provider's culture and find it difficult to trust. They would prefer a therapist from their own background. Then, too, therapists may ask questions that are banned or taboo in certain cultures.

Women of color requiring health hospitalization face great odds. They may require care for suicidal threats, for mental illness, or for a brain disorder. Often hospitalization is made under court order for purposes of protecting the client. The question of the rights of the women to refuse care is very important.

Conclusions

Although there are few specific data on the incidence and magnitude of homelessness among women of color, interest is growing among women of color themselves to learn more and to document the unique issues that face this homeless population. A review of findings indicates that some problems are gender-specific and color-specific. Because of the multiplicity of stressors, lack of access to mental health services, and general lack of knowledge of the problem, women of color seem to be more vulnerable to serious mental health problems.

RECOMMENDATIONS

The following recommendations are made with respect to health care for women of color:

1. More data should be gathered and assessments completed in order to determine extent of mental health problems for homeless women of color.

2. Attention should be directed to all areas where women of color are, such as rural areas and Indian reservations.

3. Special cultural needs of women of color must be taken into consideration when planning and providing mental health services for this population.

4. Mental health services should be accessible in all ways, including cultural.

5. Special training should be designed for mental health care providers who will provide services to women of color.

6. Special research efforts should be encouraged to determine what are effective mental health approaches to women of color.

7. Preventive measures must be taken to alleviate the pain and suffering of mentally ill women of color.

References

American Psychiatric Association. (1987). *Diagnostic and statistical manual of mental disorders* (3rd ed., rev.). Washington, DC: Author.

Anzaldua, G. (Ed.). (1990). Haciendo caras, un entrada. In *Making face, making soul* (pp. xv-xxviii). San Francisco: Aunt Lute Books.

Bassuk, E., & Rosenburg, L. (1988, July). Why does family violence occur? A case-control study. *American Journal of Public Health, 7,* 783-798.

Birch, E. L. (Ed.). (1985). *The unsheltered woman: Women and housing in the '80s.* New Jersey: Center for Urban Policy Research, Rutgers University.

Bussiere, A., Freedman, H., Menning, D., Mihaly, L., & Morales, J. (1991). Homeless women and children. *Clearing House Review* [Special issue], 431-443.

Carnicorm, G. (1982, December). The changing role of the Indian medicine man: Three case studies. *Listening Post, 4,* 21-24.

DeBruyn, L. M., Hymbaugh, K., & Valdez, N. (1988). *A community approach to suicide and violence.* Albuquerque, NM: Special Initiatives Team of Indian Health Service, Mental Health Programs Branch, Indian Health Service.

Government Accounting Office. (1977). *Returning the mentally disabled to the community: Government needs to do more.* Washington, DC: Author.

Gulati, P. (1992). Homelessness. *Journal of Sociology and Social Welfare, 19*(4).

Health Care for Homeless Information Center. (1992). *Substance abuse among homeless and low-income women: Implications for prenatal care and child development.* Washington, DC: Author.

Herman, D. B., Struening, E. L., & Barrow, S. M. (1994). Self-reported needs for help among homeless men and women. *Evaluation and Program Planning, 17,* 249-256.

Homeless Information Exchange. (1993). *Homeless families with children.* Washington, DC: National Coalition for the Homeless.

Homeless Information Exchange. (1994). *Domestic violence—A leading cause of homelessness.* Washington, DC: National Coalition for the Homeless.

Indian Health Service (IHS). (1985). Women and alcohol. *Listening Post, 5,* 41-42.

Koegel, P. (1987). *Ethnographic perspectives on homeless and homeless mentally ill women.* Washington, DC: National Institute of Mental Health.

Kunitz, S. J., Levy, J. E., & Harwood, I. A. (Ed.). (1981). *Ethnicity and medical care.* Cambridge, MA: Harvard University Press.

Lamb, R. (Ed.). (1984). *The homeless, mentally ill.* Washington, DC: American Psychiatric Association.

Liebow, E. (1993). *Tell them who I am: The lives of homeless women.* New York: Free Press.

May, P. (1987). *Suicide and suicide attempts among American Indians and Alaska natives.* Albuquerque, NM: Mental Health Programs Branch, Indian Health Service.

May, P. A., Hymbaugh, K., Aase, J. M., & Samet, J. M. (1985). Epidemiology of Fetal Alcohol Syndrome among American Indians of the Southwest. *Listening Post, 5,* 17-36.

Moraga, C., & Anzaldua, G. (Eds.). (1981). *This bridge called my back: Writing by radical women of color.* New York: Women of Color Press.

Old Dog Cross, P. (1985). Stresses encountered by American Indian women. In L. Steele (Ed.), *Medicine women.* Grand Forks, ND: INMED.

Primas, M. E. (1994, November). *The impact of homelessness on women of color.* Paper presented at the 122nd Annual Conference of the American Public Health Association.

Reissman, F., Cohen, J., & Pearl, A. (Eds.). (1964). *Mental health of the poor.* New York: Free Press.

Sullivan, W. P. (1992). Reclaiming the community: The strength, perspective, and deinstitutionalization. *Social Work, 3,* 204-209.

Watson, S. D. (1994). Minority access and health reform: A civil right to health care. *The Journal of Law, Medicine and Ethics, 22*(2), 127-136.

14 Homeless Children
A Growing and Vulnerable Population

BRENDA A. LEATH

Depending on the definition and the method of counting used, estimates of the total number of people experiencing homelessness varies from 228,000 to 600,000 a night and from 1.7 million to 3 million per year (Allen, 1994). About 25% of the current homeless population are members of homeless families—2% are married with no children, 8% are parents of children, and 15% are children (Burt, 1992). More families with children and familyless children (children who are unattached, abandoned, or disconnected from their families) are homeless today than ever before. Anecdotal evidence reveals that more families were homeless at the end of the 1980s than at the beginning, when there were virtually no shelter facilities for homeless families and no apparent demand for them, except for battered women's shelters (Burt, 1992).

On any given night, at least 100,000 children are living in emergency shelters, welfare hotels, abandoned buildings, cars, or on the streets (Institute of Medicine [IOM], 1988; National Institute on Alcohol Abuse and Alcoholism [NIAAA] and the National Institute of

Mental Health [NIMH], 1992). This figure represents the tip of the iceberg; it includes only children of intact families and not runaways, throwaways, or abandoned children on the streets or in institutions (IOM, 1988). What is more disturbing is that if current trends persist, by the turn of the century, millions of American children will have spent a portion of their childhoods without a place to call home (Mihaly, 1989).

Despite the growth of the U.S. homeless child population, difficulties persist with regard to reliably estimating this population. That is, we know that these children exist, but we are not clear about the full impact and magnitude of homelessness on our youngest and most vulnerable citizens. The 1988 findings of the Institute of Medicine's Committee on Health Care for Homeless People continues to hold true today: "Studies specifically describing the characteristics and needs of homeless children are quite sparse; studies seeking to provide an estimate of the number of homeless children nationwide are nonexistent" (IOM, 1988, p. 13).

Six years later, a review of the literature reveals continued limitations in accurately determining actual counts and profiles of the homeless population, in general, and of homeless children and youth, in particular. The use of varying definitions of homelessness, sampling techniques, and counting methodologies is the basis of this deficiency (Burt, 1992). Likewise, data on familyless youth are not exact either. Estimates suggest that 1 million youths run away from home each year, and about 25% of them become familyless street kids surviving on their own[1] (Kennedy et al., 1990; U.S. Department of Health & Human Services (DHHS) Office of the Inspector General, 1983). It is uncertain how many youth run away from institutions and other nonhome settings, or how many are spun off from homeless families (Kennedy et al., 1990).

Conservative estimates suggest that nearly 200,000 young people living in the United States are not recognized as existing. Based on counting procedures, the homeless are not *officially* counted until they reach 21 years of age (Kennedy et al., 1990; Ritter, 1989). Despite the absence of accurate estimates, most youth service programs concur that the number of adolescents who claim the streets as home is large and growing (Kennedy et al., 1990).

According to one researcher, children represent about 15% of the homeless population and are the fastest-growing subpopulation of the homeless (Burt, 1992). It is unclear to what extent familyless youth who live on the streets are included in this percentage, because the counting methods are often based on shelter users.

Although precise statistics are not available on the ethnic characteristics of homeless children, studies repeatedly show that minorities are disproportionately represented among the homeless, especially families (Burt, 1992; Shlay & Rossi, 1992; U.S. Congress, 1993; U.S. Department of Housing & Urban Development [HUD], 1994). Within the context of homeless families, over 78% of homeless adults in families are non-white (Burt, 1992). In view of the disproportionate number of homeless people of color—51% (Burt, 1992)—one might conclude that the number of homeless children of color is similarly disproportionate.

The trends just described are appalling. The United States is one of the wealthiest nations in the world, yet many of its youngest and most vulnerable citizens are falling and will fall through the cracks and add to the ranks of the homeless. This is an embarrassment and a tragedy. Prevention of child homelessness must become a national priority. Our children will inevitably assume leadership roles in carrying the nation through the 21st century and beyond. However, they can assume these roles only if they are healthy, nurtured, safe, secure, and protected and if they have access to affordable housing and health care. This holds true whether they are dependent children or surviving on their own.

The lack of a clear and comprehensive documentation process has far-reaching implications for serving these children and youth. The lack of documentation makes it difficult to assess service needs and gain clear insight into effective program designs to adequately address these children's unmet needs. Furthermore, current estimates may be grossly underreporting the actual magnitude of child homelessness. A hidden reservoir of children in desperate need of health, mental health, and other social services may exist. Overlooking this population could be tremendously costly in terms of human potential and real dollars. The long-term implications for society translate into the need to spend scarce resources for high-cost service interventions that may have been managed for far less, if this vulnerable population had been properly identified and assessed.

The size of this hidden population should be a major concern. What needs do these children have? How costly will it be to society if we wait longer before learning more about these children? How can we effectively implement primary, secondary, or tertiary preventive strategies to improve the quality of life for these children? Although homeless children present many challenges to any researcher attempting to document their existence as a result of their transient nature, we cannot continue to ignore their existence, plight, or needs.

Many shelters are currently operating at capacity. The demand for their services has grown considerably during this decade, so much, in fact, that some potential users are turned away because of inadequate space. As we attempt to document the scope of homelessness in this country, we must be mindful that counting shelter users will represent only a portion of the homeless population. Many are forced to live on the streets, in cars, in abandoned buildings, and in other places that will permit them a place to rest. In these environments, they are subjected to numerous risks and exposure to environmental elements. These elements may range from heat, cold, rain, and snow to violent perpetrators. Although they are homeless, they should have shelter and health care. A concerted effort must be made to develop methods for counting the homeless so that better systems of care can be designed to help them.

Risk Factors for Homelessness. Who are most vulnerable to homelessness? The Federal Plan to Break the Cycle of Homelessness (HUD, 1994) identifies a number of risk factors for homelessness, combining some of the macro- and microlevel factors discussed previously. Others include the following:

Poverty
Prior episodes of homelessness
Divorce or separation among men
Single parenthood among women
Leaving home or "aging out" of foster care among unattached youth
History of institutional confinement in jails, prisons, or psychiatric hospitals
Weak or overdrawn support networks of family and friends

In addition, homelessness is also a high risk to those individuals or families who are vulnerable to alcohol and substance abuse, are mentally challenged, have disabilities, have a catastrophic illness, are victims of family violence, or are unemployed or underemployed.

The Influence of Macro and Micro Factors on Homelessness Among Children and Families. How do selected variables influence homelessness? Considerable controversy exists over which factors directly cause homeless. Some researchers contend that homelessness is an outcome of structural or macrolevel influences. Others believe that personal influences are precipitating factors for homelessness that occur on the microlevel. Despite these different schools of thought, many researchers concur that homelessness is the result of a complex set of issues and factors that occur both on the macro- and microlevels. Moreover, many of these factors are interrelated and further complicate the lives of these children and families, often placing them at greater risk for short- and long-term homelessness.

The common belief is that homelessness stems from structural factors that occur on a macrolevel. These factors relate to poverty, sexism, racial bias, lack of available housing stock, imbalances between available resources and purchasing power, labor market shifts, and declining income assistance supports. Other factors occur on a microlevel and are concerned more with the individual's personal circumstances, such as health, mental health, domestic violence, alcohol or substance abuse, and disabilities. The interrelationship of these factors may serve as a precipitating influence and/or consequence of homelessness among children and their families.

Poverty. In 1992, nearly 37 million Americans were officially classified as poor (HUD, 1994; Department of Commerce, U.S. Bureau of the Census, 1993). Rates of poverty among African Americans were consistently three times higher than among whites (33% vs. 11.6% during that year). Hispanic Americans were 2.5 times more likely to be poor than whites. Not only does poverty tend to disproportionately affect ethnic groups, but it also shows a gender bias. Female-headed households are especially vulnerable to poverty. In fact, about 48.3% of female-headed households were poor in 1992—a figure that rose to about 60% for African Americans and Hispanic Americans.

During that same time period, about 22% of all children and 47% of African American children lived below the poverty line (HUD, 1994; Department of Commerce, U.S. Bureau of the Census, 1993). The lack of economic resources when the cost of living is rising places many families and children at risk of losing whatever possessions they have. The inability to pay rent or housing costs places these persons at considerable risk for homelessness.

Sexism. Gender preferences often influence the variety and number of prospective employment opportunities for women. For women with children, this phenomenon adversely affects their ability to provide adequate support for their families. Again, the absence of adequate financial resources places these families at risk of homelessness and in many cases it is a precipitating factor in homelessness. At the same time, single women with children find it more difficult to be approved for housing loans, thereby limiting their access to adequate housing in many instances. In such cases it may become difficult to avoid homelessness or to recover from it.

Racial Bias. A disproportionate number of homeless families are people of color. Although not legal, housing discrimination is not uncommon for people of color. Residential segregation on the basis of ethnicity, race (HUD, 1994; Massey & Dentin, 1993), and gender continues to exist for minorities seeking home ownership and rental opportunities. The use of "red lining" tactics may result in ineligibility for housing loans because of higher interest rates or accelerated housing costs, both circumstances that make affordable housing inaccessible to these families. Such discrimination practices encourage homelessness. Furthermore, homelessness is also encouraged when low-cost housing is available in disadvantaged neighborhoods, which are prime targets for deinvestment, abandonment, or conversion (Burt, 1992). The ability of adult family members to provide adequately for their families under such circumstances is significantly reduced.

Labor Market Changes. Shifts in the labor market from manufacturing to service-oriented jobs adversely affected many people living in both urban and rural areas. These labor market shifts left many adult family members unable to compete in the job market because of the demand for more skilled workers. Hence job prospects and opportunities shrunk for those with less education and training. Many people, in both urban and rural areas, lost their possessions and homes.

Income Assistance. Families on Aid to Families with Dependent Children (AFDC) experienced a decline in the real value of their cash benefits during the past 20 years. State-administered assistance programs were severely cut and badly eroded during the 1980s. The impact on poor families has been decreased resources and, therefore, less purchasing power. In fact, more and more AFDC families are joining the ranks of the homeless. These families don't have enough money to pay the rent and still pay for food, heat, clothing, and medical care not covered by Medicaid insurance (Ebb, Johnson, & Allen, 1989).

Family Structure. (HUD, 1994). Changes in family structure, including the growth of single-parent families, which account for 14% of all families, have also had an impact on the growth of homelessness. About 53% of African American families were headed by a single parent in 1992, as were 32% of Hispanic families. Nearly one half of African American children and two fifths of Hispanic children live in female-headed households. These increases, combined with the dearth of affordable housing, have contributed to the growth of family homelessness (Burt, 1992). These trends are likely to persist if effective interventions are not used to assist and prevent these families and children from joining the homeless rolls.

Health, Mental Health, Disabilities, Substance Abuse, and Domestic Violence. The failure to address the treatment and rehabilitation needs of people with disabilities, chronic health problems, and mental health problems has contributed to the increase in the number of people who are vulnerable to displacement and homelessness (HUD, 1994). People suffering from mental illnesses may encounter difficulties in acquiring and managing a household because of their disability. They often face inordinate challenges to acquire adequate housing and they continue to be at risk for chronic homelessness because of personal inexperience in resource management. These problems may be compounded by adverse societal influences (for example, bias).

For some families, domestic violence has been the source of housing instability. In many instances, women with children flee their homes in search of refuge and safety from life-threatening situations. They represent a subgroup of the homeless who are displaced and generally seek safety in shelters.

Substance abuse is another factor that influences homelessness. Family members with an addiction often find their resources eroding because of their need to support their addiction. Many use what limited resources they have to accomplish this. These addictions may precipitate other dynamics within the family structure and result in coexisting illnesses or domestic violence. The outcomes of these circumstances may be devastating, resulting, for example, in the disruption of the family, acquisition of HIV disease, and/or loss of housing. In contrast, some family members may resort to negative coping strategies during heightened periods of stress, including substance abuse. In such instances, recovering from homelessness may be difficult. Again, the need to use available resources to support their addictions may further disrupt their lives, and they may find it difficult to acquire and maintain adequate resources for housing.

In summary, these structural and personal factors place individuals and entire households, including the children of these families, at risk for acute and chronic homelessness. People who are burdened by severe mental illness, addiction, and potentially lethal infections, as well as those who are inexperienced in the delicate balancing act that running a household during hard times requires, are at a serious disadvantage (HUD, 1994; McChesney, 1990; Sclar, 1990; Shinn & Gillespie, 1994).

Characteristics of Homeless Children. Who are our homeless children? Several studies report the following characteristics among homeless children (Bassuk & Rosenberg, 1990).

> Some of these children are members of one- or two-parent families. The majority of these families are headed by women (Bassuk, 1990; Bassuk, Rubin, & Lauriat, 1986).
> Most of the children of these families are under age 5 (Bassuk, 1990; Bassuk & Rubin, 1987; Wright & Weber, 1987).

Children of homeless families headed by both parents appear to be more common in rural than urban areas (18% vs. 6.7%) (Patton, 1988).

The ethnic status of homeless families tends to mirror the demographic composition of the area in which they live, with Blacks and Hispanics overrepresented in cities and whites in suburban areas (Lee et al., 1990).

The majority of street children are presumed to be adolescents.

The typical assessment for street children usually reveals parental substance abuse, parental mental illness, and parental criminal activity, as well as physical, sexual, and emotional abuse (Kennedy et al., 1990).

School failure at a young age is typical for street children, which implicates unrecognized learning disorders in this group (Bassuk & Rubin, 1987; Bassuk et al., 1986; Kennedy et al., 1990).

Health Status of Homeless Children. What are some of the common health problems experienced by our children? Homeless children are perhaps one of the most vulnerable segments of our population. They have many complex needs. Among these are specific health care needs, both physical and mental. If ignored, these problems can lead to chronic or catastrophic illnesses or even death.

The following section highlights the prevalence of homelessness among children and sets forth a discussion about their health status, barriers to care, and considerations for health system reform. According to Hammen (1992), "homeless women are quintessentially stressed women" (p. 32). Many must deal with chronic stressors, eviction, domestic violence, and shelter living. As a result, they frequently feel depressed, angry, or withdrawn. As studies have shown, these chronic stressors also negatively affect those poor but housed children who are subjected to them (Longfellow & Belle 1984; Masten, 1990; Wood, Valdez, Hayashi, & Shen, 1990).

Providers who work with homeless people must face the task of reaching an isolated and often alienated population before attempting to assess the medical needs of their patients. Tasks facing providers who hope to manage the chronic health care needs of homeless people are more formidable. The challenges they face may include the following:

Identifying chronic illness
Modifying the behavior via therapy

Promoting compliance with therapy
Coordinating interventions, often with other disciplines

Women, children, youth, whole families, and older people are swelling the ranks of the homeless in many communities and cities. They bring with them a broad range of health care needs that are dramatically different from the stereotypical person on skid row or people who were deinstitutionalized from a mental health setting. This phenomenon necessitates a shift in the way health care providers understand the impact of various subpopulations or patient mix in order to design health service systems that can address their varying needs.

Many attribute homeless people's inability to adequately care for themselves to the presence of mental illness and substance abuse. However, provider attitudes, locus of care, and delivery system design all influence the outcomes of any patient encounter. A homeless person's physical attributes and perceived "value to society" may influence provider behavior and subsequently the quality of care rendered. The complex medical and social problems of the homeless exacerbate their plight in the health care arena because of the assessed financial risks to health care institutions. That is, consumption of expensive medical care related to long stays in acute care hospitals, emergency room resources, and lack of medical coverage.

The patterns of health care use by homeless people tend to be crisis-oriented rather than preventive, and the inner-city emergency room is often the most convenient point of entry into the health care system. By way of triage, the homeless person's acute bronchitis or bilateral cellulitis may not compete with a gunshot wound, appendicitis, or other severe condition needing rapid intervention. Although many of the health care problems homeless people experience could be treated in a less expensive health care setting, such as an ambulatory care clinic, their instability undermines effective treatment, compliance, and follow-up.

Children of homeless families, as well as familyless children, generally suffer from a broad range of health problems, many of which could be prevented or managed appropriately if they had proper access to primary care services. Their health problems and needs include the following (NIAAA & NIMH, 1992):

Tend to have low birth weights (Chavkin, Kristal, Seabron, & Guigli, 1987)

Suffer from poor health (Miller & Lin, 1988)

Have many common infectious illnesses such as upper respiratory tract infections (Wright, 1987; Wright et al., 1987)

Have poor access to routine health care and preventive medicine (Miller & Lin, 1988)

Are poorly nourished (Wood et al., 1990) and sometimes iron deficient (Acker, Fierman, & Dreyer, 1987)

Have elevated blood lead levels (Alperstein, Rappaport, & Flanigan, 1988)

Are often not immunized on schedule (Alperstein et al., 1988)

Are admitted to hospitals more often and frequently rely on emergency rooms for general medical care (Alperstein et al., 1988)

Have greater developmental and cognitive delays (Bassuk & Rosenberg, 1990; Molnar & Rath, 1990; Wagner & Menke, 1990; Wood et al., 1990)

Have more behavioral and emotional problems (i.e., sleep disorders, withdrawal, aggression, and short attention spans) than housed poor children (Bassuk & Rosenberg, 1990; Masten, 1990; Molnar & Rath, 1990; Whitman, Stretch, & Accardo, 1987)

Have often been thrown out of their homes because of drug use, pregnancy, gender identification, and conflicts

Homelessness affects children's health even before they are born and continues to cause damage as they develop and grow.

High-Risk Pregnancies. According to Scanlon and Brinker (1990), the estimated rate of pregnancy among homeless women is about twice the national average, with the highest pregnancy rate found among 16 to 19 year olds. A limited understanding of contraceptives, family planning services, and rape may be factors that influence this rate. In a survey conducted by the pediatric community medical staff at St. Vincent's Hospital in New York City, among children up to 18 years of age living in one SRO (single room occupancy) facility, 50% or 4 out of 8 of those biologically capable of pregnancy were pregnant. This situation has been linked with the accelerating cycle of children having children.

According to Chavin, 39% of pregnant homeless women received no prenatal care, compared to only 14% of women in low-income housing projects and 9% of the general population (NIAAA & NIMH, 1992).

The unborn child of a pregnant homeless woman is at considerable risk at the start of life because of the problems the pregnant homeless women must contend with that may interfere with obtaining medical care. Unlike pregnant women who have adequate housing, financial resources, and means of support, homeless women may be too busy finding a way to nurture, feed, and protect other children and family members to consider the unborn child until late in the pregnancy. Trying to survive on a daily basis, as well as coping with crises—abuse, eviction, and destruction of home—all influence health-seeking behaviors.

A large cohort of American adolescents and young adults have claimed the streets as their homes. Certainly the challenges of life on the street may interfere with making health seeking behavior a priority (Kennedy et al., 1990). These youth are forced to move into adolescence without the aid of a nurturing and supportive family. Survival, protection, education, nurturing, development, modeling, control, socialization, and reinforcement—all are lost or distorted when an adolescent's family is replaced with the harsh realities of the street as a home (Kennedy et al., 1990, p. 86). What replaces the nurturing process of a family is the lifestyle of the street—violence, drugs, sexual exploitation, and crime (Kennedy et al., 1990; Kufeldt & Nimmo, 1987).

Typical medical problems of street children include violent and traumatic injuries, substance abuse, sexually transmitted diseases (i.e., hepatitis and AIDS), psychiatric disturbances, skin infestations, ignored pregnancies, "unwell" babies, and common chronic illnesses exacerbated and complicated by lack of simple care (Kennedy et al., 1990).

Violence and Injuries. Violent and traumatic injuries are among the most frequent types of medical problems assessed in street children. Typical examinations reveal high incidences of gunshot and knife wounds, providing support for studies that identify homicide as the leading cause of death among young Americans (Kennedy et al., 1990). As homeless adolescents spend more time on the street, they may become more likely to perpetrate as well as be victimized by violent acts. For girls and young women on the street, violent rape is very common and often goes unreported. About half of all reported rape victims are adolescents (Flanagan & McGarrell, 1986), and a growing number are boys (Ameri-can Academy of Pediatrics [AAP], 1988).

Sexually Transmitted Diseases (STDs). Similar difficulties exist in determining the prevalence of STDs. Given the known incidence of STDs among sexually active 13 to 24 year olds, and the clinical consensus of physicians treating runaway youth, the prevalence of these infections is certainly rising. Multiple infections are quite often the rule with street children. The epidemic use of crack cocaine, the use of sex for survival, and contraction of HIV disease compound the health care needs of youths who already may have an STD. Some clinicians indicate that when HIV infection and STDs interplay, especially syphilis, a different mode of treatment, often more expensive, is required. According to some experts, syphilis becomes a different disease when it infects people who have HIV infections. Some providers feel that routine spinal taps may have to be done in order to provide effective medical care to those affected (Berry, Hooten, & Lukehart, 1987; New York State Department of Health, 1989).

HIV. Although no accurate accounting exists, many street children are infected with HIV. Their lifestyles and behaviors have serious implications for transmission among their peers. Kennedy et al. conclude, "What is known about the lifestyle of street kids, associated risks, HIV disease, and prevalence of HIV disease and STDs in the cohort, it is fairly safe to say that this segment of the population is now coendemic. The epidemiological denouement of this development has broad implications for American society profound enough to justify any and all efforts to stop its natural progression" (p. 105).

Mental Health Problems. Again, specific statistics are lacking on the magnitude of mental health problems and needs among street children. The Institute of Medicine reported that 12% of the nation's 63 million children under age 18 suffer from a mental disorder. The Institute further reports that less than half of those, or 2.5 million, were treated in 1985, leaving 5 million without care (IOM, 1988).

When describing the range of mental health problems facing these youngsters, many providers found developmental impairments, emotional disturbances characterized by states of anxiety or depression or both, and behavioral problems that led to disruptive and antisocial acts (Kennedy et al., 1990). The common findings of developmental delays, severe depression and anxiety, and learning difficulties were often experienced by children of homeless families and familyless homeless youth (Bassuk & Rubin, 1987).

Common assessments of street children seen in psychiatric consultation include the following (Kennedy et al., 1990, p. 108):

Depression, often with suicidal thoughts
Conduct disorders
Drug and alcohol abuse
  Dual diagnosis
  Sexual compulsion
Schizophrenia and drug-related psychoses
Various types of cognitive impairments
  Mental retardation
  Borderline intellectual functioning
  Drug-related delirium
  Learning disorders
  Maladaptive personality traits

Suicide. In light of epidemic adolescent suicide, suicide among street children deserves special attention ("Suicide," 1985). This group of adolescents presents all the risk factors to complete suicide. Experience on the street reveals that many suicidal attempts are successful, but they may go uninvestigated as suicide, especially if the victim is found in the midst of a drug deal or prostitution activity.

Treatment is, to say the least, challenging and often frustrating because of the lack of patient cooperation, noncompliance, mistrust, alienation, failure to continue treatment, and difficulty transferring care when the youth relocates to another community or area.

Substance Abuse. About 40% of all Americans between the ages of 25 and 30 have tried cocaine at least once (Gawin & Ellinwood, 1988). Although no official accounting of use among street children is available, the incidence of steady use is certainly higher and involves as many female as male abusers.

The influence of crack use has manifested in a variety of adverse ways with adolescent users. Such as decreased academic performance, low self-esteem, and aggressive behavior. Decreased academic performance, lowered self-esteem, and aggressive behavior are just a few examples. In fact, many studies interrelate adolescent substance abuse with parental substance abuse (Brown, 1989), a history of sexual abuse (Rohsenow, Corbet, & Devine, 1988), school failure, sexually compulsive behavior, STDs and AIDS, psychopathology, suicide (Fowler, Rich, & Young, 1986), violence, criminal activity (Marriott, 1989), prostitution (Silbert, Pines, & Lynch, 1982), child abuse (Press, 1988), and the birth of premature babies (Zuckermanet al., 1989).

As a subgroup, street children have more health care problems and more serious medical morbidities than school-based youth. Compounding these problems is the lack of access to existing health care providers. Continuity and compliance in treatment are difficult because of the transient nature of this population.

Unlike their counterparts who are enrolled in school, street children might encounter barriers to school-based clinics as a source of primary care, depending on the scope of their services and target populations. Perhaps shelter-based or linked services augmented with mobile health units would be more effective for improving access to services by street children. School-based or linked services, however, for children of homeless families who attend school may prove to be a plausible solution to address the health care needs of this group.

In summary, comprehensive research is sorely needed to investigate the magnitude of homelessness in America and to assess the health care needs of the child homeless population. Increased access to school- and shelter-based and linked services, augmented with mobile health units, should be investigated as essential components of effective service model for reaching this population. These options may prove to be less costly than care received in hospital emergency rooms.

The Need for Research and
Development of Responsive Services

Throughout this section on child homelessness, the lack of a clear definition and documentation has made it difficult to describe with certainty the special needs of this vulnerable population. Incongruent definitions of homelessness, as well as variations in sampling techniques and methodologies used to count homeless people, are major contributing factors in the dearth of reliable national data on the characteristics of the homeless population in general and children specifically.

The lack of adequate data also hampers the development of appropriate services. There are large differences in estimates of homelessness, and children are not specifically identified as individuals in most studies. Developing a coordinated system of care cannot be accomplished without a strong information base to support the foundation for service planning and development.

Research efforts should also include evaluating the effectiveness of school- and shelter-based and linked services that are augmented by mobile health units in improving access to care by homeless children. Evidence is available that shows improvements in health status and access to primary care when school-based and linked services are used by students enrolled. It would be helpful to know if similar models of care would work with homeless children. Demonstration projects would be an invaluable source of information on this topic, particularly in light of the nation's movement toward more responsive systems of care.

Considerable work has been done in the area of homelessness. However, we have only begun to scratch the surface of research, policy development, and service development. A great deal of work still lies ahead, as the nation takes greater responsibility for the well-being of its youngest and most vulnerable citizens.

Recommendations/ Considerations for Health Care Reform

On the basis of the findings discussed in this section, the following recommendations are being made to improve the manner in which services are developed and provided for homeless children.

1. Conduct a national study on homeless children and street children to document their existence, health status, and health needs.

2. Support demonstration projects that determine which innovative models or systems of care are most effective for use among homeless and street children.

3. Develop a uniform definition for homeless children, incorporating language that is applicable to street children and facilitates the use of a uniform process for collecting information.

4. Develop guidelines that will encourage the use of AIDS educators and counselors in clinical settings that target homeless youth to assist in keeping the majority of those patients who are still uninfected from becoming so.

5. Develop strategies that put adequate resources in place, test those at risk, treat infected patients, and protect the patients who are still uninfected.

6. Conduct research on homeless children, employing a systems approach to investigate macro- and microlevel influences on the development of homeless children.

7. Support innovative service delivery models to include school-based or linked and shelter-based or linked services.

8. Establish a coordinated, preventive, and long-term network or system of care for homeless children or youth.

9. Design research efforts to better understand the nature, extent, and severity of the problem of family homelessness by implementing the following:

   a. Develop reliable estimates of the incidence and prevalence of family homelessness that examine variations across geographic locales, urban and rural sites, and racial groups.

   b. Develop a system of monitoring that can assess changes in the prevalence of homelessness over time.

   c. Investigate how the experience of family homelessness varies as a function of the cause for homelessness—natural disaster versus domestic dispute versus eviction.

   d. Reassess the role of the public health nurse in the delivery of community-based services to the homeless population.

   e. Incorporate greater flexibility in the eligibility requirements for homeless families and children to receive entitlement benefits.

   f. Develop policies and incentive programs that are designed to increase the number of providers trained to work with homeless populations.

   g. Include cultural sensitivity, as well as training geared to the homeless, in the curricula of health and social service professionals.

h. Require residency training experiences and internships within the homeless population.

Note

1. Throwaways are defined as children and adolescents who are evicted from their homes by their parents or another adult in a position of responsibility for them.

References

Acker, P. J., Fierman, A. H., & Dreyer, B. P. (1987). An assessment of parameters of health care and nutrition in homeless children (abs.). *American Journal of Disabled Children, 141,* 388

Allen, M. (1994). "Children and families in crisis" and "Housing and Homelessness" in *The State of America's Children: Yearbook, 1994.* Washington, DC: Children's Defense Fund.

Alperstein, G., Rappaport C., & Flanigan, J. M. (1988). Health problems of homeless children in New York City. *American Journal of Public Health, 78,* 1232-1233.

American Academy of Pediatrics Committee on Adolescence. (1988). American Academy of Pediatrics Committee states: Rape and the adolescent. *Pediatrics, 81*(4), 595-597.

Bassuk, E. L. (1990). The problem of family homelessness. In E. L. Bassuk, R. W. Carman, & L. F. Weinrab, (Eds.), with M. M. Herzig *Community care for homeless families: A program design manual* (pp. 7-12). Washington, DC: Interagency Council on the Homeless.

Bassuk, E. L., & Rosenberg, L. (1990). Psychological characteristics of homeless children and children with homes. *Pediatrics, 85,* 257-261.

Bassuk, E. L., & Rubin, L. (1987). Homeless children: A neglected population. *American Journal of Orthopsychiatry, 57,* 279-286.

Bassuk, E. L., Rubin, L., & Lauriat, A. (1986). Characteristics of homeless families. *American Journal of Public Health, 76,* 1097-1101.

Berry, C. D., Hooten, T. M., & Lukehart, S. A. (1987). Medical intelligence: Neurologic relapse after benzathine penicillin therapy for secondary syphilis in a patient with HIV infection. *New England Journal of Medicine, 316*(25), 1587-1589.

Brown, S. A. (1989). Life events of adolescents in relation to personal and parental substance abuse. *American Journal of Psychiatry, 146*(4), 484-489.

Burt, M. R. (1992). *Over the edge: The growth of homelessness in the 1980s.* New York: Russell Sage Foundation.

Chavkin, W., Kristal, A., Seabron, C., & Guigli, P. E. (1987). The reproductive experience of women living in hotels for the homeless in New York City. *New York State Journal of Medicine, 87,* 10-13.

Department of Commerce, U.S. Bureau of the Census (1993).

Ebb, N., Johnson, C., & Allen, M. (1989). Family income. In *A vision for America's future: An agenda for the 1990s.* Washington, DC: Children's Defense Fund.

Flanagan, T. J., & McGarrell, E. F. (Eds.). (1986). *Sourcebook of criminal justice statistics, 1985*. Washington, DC: U.S. Department of Justice, Bureau of Justice Statistics.

Fowler, R. C., Rich, C. L., & Young, D. (1986). San Diego suicide study. II. Substance abuse in young cases. *Archives of General Psychiatry, 43*(10), 962-965.

Gawin, F. H., & Ellinwood, E. H. (1988). Cocaine and other stimulants: Actions, abuse, and treatment. *New England Journal of Medicine, 318*(18), 1173-1182.

Hammen, C. (1992). Parenting. In National Institute on Alcohol Abuse and Alcoholism and the National Institute of Mental Health (Eds.), *Homeless families with children: Research perspectives* (Publication No. (ADM) 92-1848, pp. 15-26). Rockville, MD: U.S. Department of Health and Human Services.

Institute of Medicine. (1988). *Homelessness, health, and human needs*. Washington, DC: National Academy Press.

Kennedy, J. T., Petrone, J., Deisher, R. W., Emerson, J., Heslop, P., Bastible, D., & Arkovitz, M. (1990). Health care for familyless, runaway street kids. In P. W. Brickner, L. K. Scharer, B. A. Conanan, M. Savarese, & B. C. Scanlan (Eds.), *Under the safety net: The health and social welfare of the homeless in the United States* (pp. 82-117). New York: Norton.

Kufeldt, K., & Nimmo, M. (1987). Youth on the street: Abuse and neglect in the eighties. *Childhood Abuse & Neglect, 11*(4), 531-543.

Lee, M. A., Haught, K., Redlener, I., Fant, A., Fox, E., & Somers, S. A. (1990). Health care for children in homeless families. In P. W. Brickner, L. K. Scharer, B. A. Conanan, M. Savarese, & B. C. Scanlan (Eds.), *Under the safety net: The health and social welfare of the homeless in the United States* (pp. 119-138). New York: Norton.

Longfellow, C., & Belle, D. (1984). Stressful environments and their impact on children. In J. Humphrey (Ed.), *Stress in childhood* (pp. 63-78). New York: AMS.

Marriott, M. (1989, February 20). After 3 years, crack plague only gets worse. *New York Times*, p. A1.

Massey, D. S., & Denton, N. A. (1993). *American apartheid: Segregation and the making of the underclass*. Cambridge, MA: Harvard University Press.

Masten, A. S. (1990). *Homeless children: Risk, trauma, and adjustment*. Paper preented at the annual meeting of the American Psychological Association, Boston, MA.

McChesney, K. Y. (1990). Family homelessness. *Journal of Social Issues, 46*, 191-205.

Mihaly, L. (1989). Homelessness and housing. In *A vision for America's future: An agenda for the 1990s* (pp. 27-36). Washington, DC: Children's Defense Fund.

Miller, D. S., & Lin, E. H. B. (1988). Children in sheltered homeless families: Reported health status and use of health services. *Pediatrics, 81*(5), 668-673.

Molnar, J. M., & Rath, W. R. (1990). *Beginning at the beginning: Public policy and homeless children*. Paper presented at the annual meeting of the American Psychological Association, Boston, MA.

National Institute on Alcohol Abuse and Alcoholism and the National Institute of Mental Health. (1992). *Homeless families with children: Research perspectives* (Publication No. (ADM) 92-1848). Rockville, MD: U.S. Department of Health and Human Services.

New York State Department of Health. (1989). *Recommendations for diagnosing and treating syphilis in human immunodeficiency virus infected patients* (Series 89-65). Albany: Author.

Patton, L. T. (1988). The rural homeless. In Institute of Medicine (Ed.), *Homelessness, health, and human needs* (pp. 183-217). Washington, DC: National Academy Press.

Press, S. (1988). Crack and fatal child abuse. *Journal of the American Medical Association, 260*(21), 3132.

Ritter, B. (1989). Abuse of the adolescent. *New York State Journal of Medicine, 89,* 156-158.

Rohsenow, D. J., Corbet, R., & Devine, D. (1988). Molested as children: A hidden contribution to substance abuse? *Journal of Substance Abuse Treatment, 5*(1), 13-18.

Scanlan, B. C., & Brickner, P. W. (1990). Clinical concerns in the care of homeless persons. In P. W. Brickner, L. K. Scharer, B. A. Conanan, & B. C. Scanlan (Eds.), *Under the safety net: The health and social welfare of the homeless in the United States* (pp. 69-81). New York: W. W. Norton.

Sclar, E. (1990). Homeless and housing policy. *American Journal of Public Health, 80,* 1039-1040.

Shinn, M., & Gillespie, C. (1994). The roles of housing and poverty in the origins of homelessness. *American Behavioral Scientist, 37,* 505-521.

Shlay, A. B., & Rossi, P. (1992). Social science research and contemporary studies of homelessness. *Annual Review of Sociology, 18,* 129-160.

Silbert, M. H., Pines, A. M., & Lynch, T. (1982). Substance abuse and prostitution. *Journal of Psychoactive Drugs, 14*(3), 193-197.

Suicide—United States, 1970-1980. (1985). *Morbidity and Mortality Weekly Report, 34*(24), 353-357.

U.S. Congress. (1993). *1993 Green Book* (House of Representatives, Committee on Ways and Means). Washington, DC: Government Printing Office.

U.S. Department of Health & Human Services, Office of the Inspector General, Region X. (1983). *Runaway and homeless youth: National program inspection.* Washington, DC: Author.

U.S. Department of Housing & Urban Development. (1994). *Priority: Home! The federal plan to break the cycle of homelessness* (Publication No. HUD-1454-CPD). Washington, DC: Author.

Wagner, J., & Menke, E. (1990). *The mental health of homeless children.* Paper presented at the annual meeting of the American Public Health Association, New York.

Whitman, H. Y., Stretch, J., & Accardo, P. (1987). *The crisis in homelessness: Effects on children and families* (Testimony presented before the U.S. House of Representatives Select Committee on Children, Youth, and Families). Washington, DC: Government Printing Office.

Wood, D. L., Valdez, R. B., Hayashi, T., & Shen, A. (1990). Health of homeless children and housed poor children. *Pediatrics, 86,* 858-866.

Wright, J. D. (1987). The National Center for the Homeless program. In R. D. Bingham, R. E. Green, & S. B. White (Eds.), *The homeless in contemporary society* (pp. 150-169). Newbury Park, CA: Sage.

Wright, J. D., & Weber, E. (1987). *Homelessness and health.* New York: McGraw-Hill.

Wright, J. D., Weber-Burdin, E., Knight, J., & Lam, J. (1987). *The National Health Care for the Homeless program: The first year.* Amherst: University of Massachusetts.

Zuckerman, B., Frank, D. A., Hingson, R., Amaro, H., Levenson, S. M., Kayne, H., Parker, S., Vinci, R., Aboagye, K., Fried, L. E., Cabral, H., Timperi, R., & Bauchner, H. (1989). Original article: Effects of maternal marijuana and cocaine use on fetal growth. *New England Journal of Medicine, 320*(12), 762-768.

15 Ethical Issues in Research

MARIAN GRAY SECUNDY

A broad range of issues can be covered under the rubric of ethical issues in research as they relate to women of color. However, specific concerns relative to issues of inequality, inclusion/exclusion, and informed consent are of most significance, in my opinion. In examining situations in which these issues surface, it is important to remember the real ways these issues reflect and represent the moral fabric of our lives, because ethical concerns are about just that—the moral fabric of our lives. When we focus on ethical issues in medicine, biotechnology, philosophy, and theology, we are attempting to identify, examine, and analyze that which we believe to be good and right about the environment or the society in which we live. Elkins and Brown (1993) observed in a recent article that "from a societal perspective, ethical reflection on health care issues focuses on the continued liberty of citizens when they are patients and on the fair distribution of resources" (p. 31). Describing the views of ethicist physician Edmund Pellegrino, Abrams (1993) states that "ethics governs our finer, hour-by-hour activity, our more intimate behavior. . . . Ethics implies trust" (p. 27). Certain principles govern Western civilization's notions of the good and the right. We aspire to these principles, but we pay them lip service in our attempts to provide health care and to enhance our knowledge about the health status of our citizenry. Our failure to fulfill these aspirations is the problem I address.

In our failures to provide adequate care to all Americans, we have been most remiss in helping the poor, minorities, and women, particularly women of color. We have failed to develop a knowledge base of sufficient quality to improve our preventive, primary care, and tertiary care services to these populations. Women of color particularly have been neglected; they have not been allowed to function or to participate as equal partners in analyzing or evaluating their own environments. We find the consequences of this neglect in the grim demographics that describe the state of women's health and in a variety of problems relative to diagnoses, management/treatment, and research.

Women are more susceptible than men to disease, have a worse overall health status than men, have greater prevalence of certain health problems, and respond differently when confronted with certain health problems than do men. Specific areas of concern for women's health are cardiovascular disease, cancer, diabetes, AIDS, substance abuse, depression, effects of stress, violence/battery/rape, aging, and poverty. National statistics and data are almost nonexistent for Hispanic/Latino women, Asian/Pacific Islander women, and Native American women. They, however, have many of the same problems that we see confronting African American women, specifically lower life expectancy (compared to white women), poverty, and increased vulnerability to mental health disorders. Black women are contracting AIDS at rates three times faster than whites. Black women are at greater risk for being homicide victims and victims of violence than are white women. Substance abuse is almost three times more prevalent among Black women, compared to white peers, and Black women are more likely to suffer relapses. There are more deaths from breast cancer, higher incidences of gonorrhea and syphilis, and greater limitations upon physical functioning earlier in life than white women experience. Women of color also obtain less prenatal care, have greater maternal mortality, and lose children in infancy at higher rates than do white women. Black women also die more frequently and sooner of hypertension and cardiovascular disease (American Cancer Society, 1990; Plicta, 1992, p. 155; White, 1990, p. xv).

Angela Davis (1990) comments,

> We have become cognizant of the urgency of contextualizing Black women's health in relation to the prevailing political conditions, while our health is undeniably assaulted by natural forces frequently beyond our control. All too often the enemies of our physical and emotional well-being are social and political. (p. 19)
>
> The major barrier to Black Women's Health is poverty. Poverty increases vulnerability. . . . Standing at the intersection of racism, sexism, and economic injustice, Black women have been compelled to bear the brunt of this complex oppressive process." (p. 21)

A growing number of vibrant Black women are being devastated by a multitude of physical and emotional ailments. A downward trend in their health has occurred at a time when this country has developed state of the art medical technology that is envied around the world (White, 1990, p. xiv). Of particular concern is the damaged mental and physical health of Black women. Adisa (1990) noted that

> studies show that stress is linked to several physical and emotional problems that disproportionately affect Black women, including heart disease, depression, ulcers, hypertension, and drug and alcohol abuse. (p. 11)
>
> I don't know one Black woman, regardless of educational status, economic condition, or social position, who is not faced with stress. Some people think stress is like the blues, but it's not. Blues is medicine. . . . The blues heals. . . . Stress doesn't do that. Stress does not heal; it infects; it's only satisfied when you're dead. It is the venom that gets into all Black women's blood, causing our bodies to swell and explode, extinguishing our lives. (p. 12)
>
> Did you ever wonder why so many sisters look so angry? Why we walk like we've got bricks in our bags and will slash and curse you at the drop of a hat? It's because stress is hemmed into our dresses, pressed into our hair, mixed into our perfume, and painted on our fingers. Stress from the broken promises, the blatant lies; stress from always being at the bottom. (p. 14)

The reality for women of color is that they are victims of a health care system that is unequal, lacking in equity, exclusionary, and often inadequate in securing appropriate informed consent when women are included. All levels of the health care enterprise are affected. Problems exist in relation to direct service as well as in areas of research at public and private levels.

Unequal Access to Care

Despite the availability of health care and research projects, women of color often do not have adequate access to that health care or to those research projects. Poverty is a major factor in limiting access. Compromised health status due to poor nutrition, substandard housing, insufficient clothing, and improper sanitation is not a problem for Third World countries only but exists here as well. Health researchers have described significant disparities in the use of major diagnostic and therapeutic interventions for women, compared with their use for men. Women reportedly are more likely than men to use health services, but they are also more likely to encounter financial barriers to care (Plicta, 1992). The Clinton health task force was cognizant of the approximately 14 million women of childbearing age who remain without insurance coverage and the 5 million who have insurance that excludes coverage for prenatal care and delivery. Efforts were made to propose suitable coverage for all. Women of color who were poor continue to be less likely to have had Pap smears or breast examinations. In the case of all women, older ones were less likely than younger women to have received preventive care of any kind (Clancy & Massion, 1992, p. 1918). The problems described are compounded because of lack of adequate documentation and too few surveys and databases that delineate the facts.

Unequal Research Treatment

Most biomedical studies have used men as models for the prototypical study population, with subsequent results applied to women as though such diseases or conditions would have the same natural history of response (Pinn, 1992a, p. 1921). This is indeed an erroneous assumption. Less is understood about the health of women because of the nature of the limitations of the research generated about them. The significant exclusion of women as research subjects has resulted in incomplete data and inadequate information about women's health generally and specifically.

Fortunately, current federal initiatives that focus on women's health are aimed at correcting the existing inequality. The Women's Health Initiative of the National Institutes of Health and the work of the MEDTEP Research Centers on Minority Populations are encouraging. For example, the goals of the NIH Women's Health Initiative are described as follows:

> Address inequities in women's health research
> Ensure that women are included in clinical studies
> Identify gaps in knowledge about women's health
> Establish a comprehensive research agenda for women's health
> Assist in funding priorities
> Create collaborative efforts of the scientific community, extramural community, advocacy groups, and the health industry
> Look at the health of women through all the stages of their lives
> Integrate basic sciences, clinical trials, and new technologies

MEDTEP research centers across the country are designed to support patient outcomes research, provide technical assistance and research training, and disseminate information, with the intent of improving the appropriateness and effectiveness of health care services to minority patients, including women of color. New research findings resulting from this work may help in developing appropriate clinical strategies that provide the most effective care for minority populations and in the formulation of related policy issues (Adams, 1993).

Informed Consent

When one considers the ethical issues inherent in enabling informed consent for women in research trials and in therapeutic interventions, one is reminded of the historical imbalances of power. Elkins and Brown (1993, p. 33) speak of those situations in which women's freedom has been diminished or made unstable. As investigators struggle with newly defined obligations to communicate and to include women and women of color, they are singularly disadvantaged by not having had previous experience or training in addressing these challenges. Charged with informing women of their options and alternatives and of the specific nature of a particular study and its risk and discomforts, investigators must learn to do so in an atmosphere devoid of external coercion, manipulation, and infringement of bodily integrity. Elkins and Brown also have observed that "the practice of informed consent . . . is applicable to clinical cases in which the woman involved has the ability and the opportunity to read, has social advantage, and has significant economic power. . . . [It] has little relevance for physicians facing . . . decisions involving patients who do not bring such privileges" (p. 32).

I agree that the better educated woman is at an advantage, but I do not agree that informed consent is irrelevant to the less advantaged. A limited educational background does not imply stupidity. The burden is upon the investigator and the clinician to find effective ways to communicate. We acknowledge that some limitations may modify or mitigate the obligation of informed consent, for example, emergency illnesses, but as Heland (1993) says, "any compromise or relaxation of the full ethical obligation of informed consent requires special ethical justification" (p. 2224). Respect for people requires that an effort be made. Society must rid itself of notions that women's informational and reasoning capacities are limited. However, a rich opportunity does exist to explore whether and how gender differences may be reflected in the way women conceptualize their experience of illness, the meanings attached to such experiences, and interpretations of those experiences by others. We must continue to ask if there are morally relevant differences between men and women. Respect for individuals carries with it notions of autonomy. Being autonomous means having the capacity to choose and participate in setting one's own agenda. Informed consent is not an end but a means, not an act but a process. What is encouraged and necessary is the development of a relationship between physician/investigator and patient.

"Freedom is maximized in relationships of trust, understanding is enhanced in the nuanced frameworks of conversation . . . situated in relationships of mutuality of respect and . . . equality of personal power" (American College of Obstetricians and Gynecologists, 1993, p. 4).

Federal officials claim that

> by the year 2000, women's health should be an integral part of the scientific mainstream, with gender disparities in research programs relegated to historical interest. No longer will excuses which have contributed to some of the inequities and inequalities described above be acceptable for we will have moved away from an era of exclusion to one of inclusion. (Pinn, 1992b, p. 1921)

Inclusion/Exclusion

The move toward inclusion of women in all aspects of clinical research is long overdue. No longer can women be excluded, based on rationalizations, such as the possibility that cyclical hormonal changes may confound research results; the increased costs of studies that include sex-specific hypotheses or subgroup analyses; or difficulties of recruitment. Exclusion is now appropriately acknowledged as unethical. Women cannot gain from new advances in therapy and interventions if they are not included in clinical trials that assess safety and efficacy. Pinn (1992a) has commented that "the health care system must provide medical care based upon sufficient understanding of sex differences and the influences of hormones on health and disease. Scientists, practitioners, patients, and the public, of both sexes, must be sensitized about the need, value, and benefits of such directed research" (p. 327).

Dresser (1992) has observed that exclusion is a glaring moral mistake and that heretofore NIH and other scientific research agencies have had an ethical blind spot. To date, physicians lack adequate evidence on whether women and people of color will be helped, harmed, or not affected at all by numerous therapies (pp. 24-25). In much basic research, even female rats have frequently been excluded as research subjects. Recent findings that aspirin can help prevent migraine headaches are based on data from males only, even though women suffer from migraine up to three times as often as men. A study of the relationship between caffeine and heart disease involved 45,000 research subjects, all of them male. Dresser noted that even a pilot project on the impact of obesity on breast and uterine cancer was conducted solely on men (p. 24). Keeping in mind principles of beneficence, biomedical research should be designed to maximize benefit and minimize harm, Dresser reminds us.

"White males only" research withholds benefits from other groups and exposes women to risk when they follow recommendations based only on data from white males. When diseases that affect women and people of color are given low funding priority, knowledge that could alter current ineffective or detrimental routine medical care is never produced. Clearly, as we have learned, simple extrapolation from white males to everyone else can be dangerous (Dresser, 1992):

> Scientists and policy makers must recognize that the choice is not whether to protect women and people of color from research risks. Instead, the choice is whether to expose some consenting members of these groups to risk in the closely monitored research setting, or to expose many more of them to risk in the clinical setting without these safeguards. (p. 27)

Appropriate guidelines can and must be established to maximize protection of female subjects.

When speaking of beneficence, ethicists are addressing issues that focus on the importance of demonstrating a concern for the welfare of all and/or a concern for the welfare of a particular individual. An extremely important principle in medicine and health care, beneficence, requires attention to issues of efficacy, safety, and justice in distribution of care and in efforts to obtain new knowledge through research strategies. Justice/fairness as a concept to which we pay allegiance requires attention to issues of fair distribution of the benefits and burdens of biomedical research. Within the context of patient care, the concept would have us address issues of allocation of resources and equitable ways in which we can make such allocations, keeping in mind the critical importance of standards of adequacy and quality of care to all.

Heretofore, taxpayers who have been excluded from study populations are in fact paying for research without assurances that they
will share in any health benefits these studies might produce. Inclusion in research presents potential dangers of its own to disadvantaged and minority populations, however. The careless disregard
for human life and health manifested, for example, in the notor-
ious Tuskegee study is an ever-present reminder that inclusion
without guidelines, sanctions, and constant vigilance is not enough
(Jones, 1993).

Intentional or not, exclusionary practices reflect implicit social
worth judgments as to who ought to have priority in obtaining the
fruits of biomedical research. Further, as Dresser (1992) observes, "The
choice of which differences 'matter' inevitably reflects and reinforces
existing social structures and normality" (p. 27). An expansion of the
disease model of health is also essential if we are to maximize chances
of avoiding stereotypical research findings. We must protect against
discriminatory use of findings about women of color. Diversity must
be acknowledged, recognized, and appreciated. A more interactive
model of research is needed to foster dialogue between researchers
of different disciplines, biomedical, psychosocial, and behavioral,
and between researchers and community (Elkins & Brown, 1993, p.
32). Our reading of Minow (1990, pp. 29-74) suggests that she sees
the goal as movement beyond the restrictive traditional patterns of
labeling difference toward a richer more expansive view. Analysis
of diversity is not sufficient, however. Clearly, diversity in decision
making must occur to allow for greater inclusion of women and,
specifically, women of color.

Inclusion is meaningless if uninformed and/or coerced. Participants in research should share in the decision making regarding their
own health care; this is of critical importance. Autonomy as an ethical
construct provides the rationale and framework for informed consent.

Summary

As attempts are made to ensure health care reforms, advocates for
women of color must attend carefully to the mechanisms by which

problems of unequal access, unequal research treatment, inclusion, and informed consent can be corrected and/or improved. Insofar as such corrections and/or improvements are made for all, they will inevitably affect women in more positive ways. However, a specific woman's agenda for research and attention to health care needs is necessary and ought to be combined with similar focus and attention to minority populations across the board. Caregivers, investigators, and patients all have duties and responsibilities in this regard. We can improve the moral fabric of women's lives—and truly of all our lives—if we attend to the task with commitment and diligence.

A policy report based on a 1993 survey conducted for the Commonwealth Fund Commission on Women's Health, New York City ("Ensuring Affordable," 1994) set forth seven goals for health care reform. These are clear and straightforward, designed to address problems of unequal access to care, unequal research treatment, inclusion, and informed consent. Commitment on the part of all is of vital significance to an ethical agenda for women's health and research about women's health status and their need for the following:

Affordable coverage for all Americans

Benefits that cover services essential to women's health

Cost sharing at levels that are realistic for low-income women and their families

Programs that expand the availability of primary care and other essential services in under-served communities and provide support services that women need to enable them to obtain health care

Payment rates for public programs that do not jeopardize access to care for women who depend on Medicare and Medicaid

A requirement that plans and providers provide information on performance, quality, consumer satisfaction, and cost

Provisions that promote medical innovations and research about health care problems for women and men

The evident interdependence of a meaningful research agenda and health care reforms in service delivery and coverage cannot be overestimated. Without such innovations and improvements in delivery and coverage, it is unlikely that issues of equity, equality, inclusion, and informed consent can ever be resolved.

References

Abrams, F. R. (1993). Commentary on ACOG Committee Opinion #108 May 1992, Ethical Dimensions of Informed Consent. *Women's Health Issues, 3*(1), 27-28.

Adams, D. L. (1993, April). *MEDTEP research centers on minority populations.* Document prepared in conjunction with the Center for Medical Effectiveness Research, Special Populations Study Group of the AHCPR for Prevention '93, St. Louis, MO.

Adisa, O. P. (1990). Rocking in the sun light: Stress and Black women. In E. C. White (Ed.), *The Black women's health book* (pp. 11-14). Seattle: The Seal Press.

American Cancer Society. (1990). *Career facts and figures.* Washington, DC. Author.

American College of Obstetricians and Gynecologists. (1993). Ethical dimensions of informed consent: Statement of the American College of Obstetricians and Gynecologists. *Women's Health Issues, 3*(l), p. 4.

Clancy, C., & Massion, C. T. (1992). American women's health care: A patchwork quilt with gaps. *Journal of the American Medical Association, 268*(14), 1918-1920.

Davis, A. Y. (1990). Sick and tired of being sick and tired: The politics of Black women's health. In E. C. White (Ed.), *The Black women's health book* (pp. 18-26). Seattle: The Seal Press.

Dresser, R. (1992, January-February). Wanted: Single white male for medical research. *Hastings Center Report*, pp. 24-29.

Elkins, T., & Brown, D. (1993). Informed consent: Commentary on the ACOG Ethics Committee statement. *Women's Health Issues, 3*(l), 31-33.

Ensuring affordable health care for women. (1994, September 19). *AHA News*, p. 6.

Heland, K. (1993). Ethics versus law: A lawyer's road map to the Ethics Committee opinion on informed consent [Commentary]. *Women's Health Issues, 3*(1), 22-24.

Jones, J. (1993). *Bad blood: The Tuskegee syphillis experiment.* New York: Free Press.

Minow, M. (1990). *Making all the difference: Inclusion, exclusion, and American law.* Ithaca, NY: Cornell University Press.

Pinn, V. (1992a). Commentary: Women, research, and the National Institutes of Health. *American Journal of Preventive Medicine, 8*(5), 324-327.

Pinn, V. (1992b). Women's health research: Prescribing change and addressing the issues [Editorial]. *Journal of the American Medical Association, 268*, 1921-1922.

Plicta, S. (1992). The effects of woman abuse. *Women's Health Institute, 2*(3), 154-169.

White, E. C. (1990). Introduction. In E. C. White (Ed.), *The Black women's health book* (pp. i-xv). Seattle: The Seal Press.

16 Conclusion

DAVID R. WILLIAMS

NIKI DICKERSON

The health needs of an invisible U.S. population are being ignored. Women make up over half of the U.S. population, and women of color are becoming a larger proportion of the population of women. The preceding chapters emphasize the unique experiences of women of color in the United States. They provide eloquent testimony to the fact that these populations are characterized by considerable diversity in sociodemographic characteristics, as well as in the distribution of disease and risk factors for disease. Although the health problems of women of color overlap with those of women in general, and there are some commonalities to the health issues faced by minority women in general, there is some distinctiveness to the health profile of each major subgroup of women of color, and these health problems can be understood and effectively addressed only within their unique context.

Research Implications

Understanding this distinctiveness and diversity is contingent on adequate description of the health status of each group. One of the disturbing themes permeating all of the contributions to this volume is the pathetic paucity of adequate data on the health of women in general, and women of color in particular. Little is known about the distribution of specific diseases in the diverse groups that make up the Hispanic category, the Asian Pacific Islander American (APIA) population, and the hundreds of tribal groups that make up the American Indian population.

There is a long history of inattention to and marginalization of the health care needs of women in general (Scully, 1980). The marginal and powerless status of women of color in American society exacerbates this general pattern. In addition, the unavailability of data for women of color reflects the politics of racial categorization in the United States and the limitations of our current approaches. The Office of Management and Budget's Directive 15 requires all federal statistical agencies to report racial data by four racial groups (White, Black, American Indian or Alaskan Native, and Asian or Pacific Islander) and one ethnic category (Hispanic). These categories combine biologically oriented notions about race with notions of nationality, ethnicity, and cultural identification in ways that lack coherence, consistency, and usefulness. Currently the federal health statistic system provides little data on Arab Middle Eastern American women because people from North Africa and the Middle East are categorized as White; although the White population contains a broad range of ethnic groups that have distinctive histories and cultures, little attention is paid to exploring ethnic variations in the non-Hispanic White population.

For most of this century, the contrast between whites and non-whites (a category that consisted almost exclusively of blacks) was the major basis of racial differentiation in the reporting of health status. However, despite a recent and welcome emphasis on collecting more data on the racial and ethnic minority populations that make up a growing proportion of the American population, inadequate attention is given to the nontrivial cultural differences that exist for subgroups within each of the major racial populations. The use of pooled data for a particular racial category, such as Hispanic or APIA American, can produce results that are misleading and that lead to the neglect of serious health problems within specific subgroups of those populations. The federal government is currently engaged in a process of reviewing and evaluating the current system of racial classification. It is critically important that the new classification system give greater attention to identifying the broad range of cultural and national origin variation within the American population. Identifiers for these racial and ethnic groups should be included in federal, state, and local health data collection systems.

Historically, the study of racial differences in health in the United States has been driven by an ideological orientation that views race as capturing biological differences between human population groups (Krieger, 1987). This biological view of race is not supported by scientific evidence, and the extant racial categories do not capture biological distinctiveness (Cooper, 1984; Williams, Lavizzo-Mourey, & Warren, 1994). Racial groups are more alike than different in terms of biological characteristics, and genetic and scientific criteria for assigning individuals to one particular racial group versus another do not exist. Thus, biological approaches and models are likely to make a very limited contribution to identifying and understanding health status variations for women of color. Moreover, when biological variables emerge as important, they are likely to operate by interacting with environmental ones.

Much of the current research on racial differences in disease conducted by the National Institutes of Health continues to emphasize biological differences. Biological explanations tend to focus on factors within the individual and to develop solutions that target individuals. Thus, a preoccupation with the biological sources of racial variations in health can effectively divert attention from the current societal arrangements and policies that affect the health status of women of color (Williams et al., 1994). Science is not value-free, and one important way that larger cultural ideology and political interests shape research is by determining which research questions get asked and which projects get funded (Duster, 1984). Thus, as the research agenda on the health of women of color develops, it will be important to give biological hypotheses the scientific attention and financial support commensurate with their likely contribution to understanding racial and ethnic variations in health.

In contrast to the biological view, the contributors to this volume consistently emphasize that the social context of women of color gives rise to the particular patterns of disease evident within these populations. They indicate that the health outcomes of women are linked not just to individual deficits or cultural pathology but to the social location of women in society. They emphasize the need to identify the systemic processes and forces that create the health problems that women face.

Race and ethnic status is a crude indicator of distinctive histories and specific living conditions of particular social groups. Research that gives more explicit attention to the ways in which social, economic, and political forces constrain the lives of women of color can enhance our understanding of the determinants of their health problems and the intervention strategies required to address them. Several contributors to this volume note that socioeconomic status (SES) is an important construct that deserves more research attention. Low SES is associated with poor living conditions, exposure to high levels of stress, and inadequate access to quality medical care. SES is one of the strongest and most pervasive predictors of variations in health outcomes (Adler et al. 1994; Bunker, Gomby, & Kehrer, 1989; Williams, 1990). People of low social status have higher rates of death, disease, and disability than their higher SES counterparts. The importance of understanding the role of low SES is highlighted by the fact that both income inequality and SES disparities in health have increased in recent years. In addition, there is a disturbing trend toward widening of racial differentials in health for both males and females (Williams & Collins, 1995).

Tom-Orme (Chapter 3, this volume) noted that changes in the lifestyle of Native American women—increased sedentary behavior and greater consumption of high-fat foods—have probably played an important role in the high rate of diabetes in that population. These risk factors for diabetes are examples of variables that are too frequently viewed only at the psychological level. It is important for researchers and practitioners to recognize that health behaviors are best understood and effectively modified only in context of the social conditions that initiate and maintain them. Large-scale historical and economic forces combine to determine the production and marketing of particular food products to vulnerable populations (Maxwell & Jacobson, 1989). More generally, contributors to this volume have illustrated that large-scale changes in the U.S. and global economies, as well as in social and economic conditions in host countries, can all have significant effects on the health of subgroups of U.S. women of color.

Greater attention to understanding the role of acculturation in health can also enhance our knowledge of the health status of women of color. There has been some research attention recently to the potential protective effects of host cultures (Vega & Amaro, 1994), and there is interest in identifying the particular cultural symbols, attitudes, or experiences that may account for the superior health status of some immigrant groups, such as Mexican American women (James, 1993). However, Zambrana and Ellis (Chapter 4, this volume) emphasize that acculturation is a multi-dimensional process that may have both positive and adverse effects on particular health outcomes. More attention needs to be given to delineating both the health-enhancing and the stress-producing aspects of acculturation and to identifying the ways in which they interact with socioeconomic status and other risk factors to affect health and well-being.

As noted by several contributors to this volume, another important but neglected factor affecting the health status of women of color is racism. A small but growing body of evidence suggests that racism may be an important determinant of the health status of populations of color in the United States (Cooper, 1993; Krieger, Rowley, Herman, Avery, & Phillips, 1993; Williams, in press; Williams et al., 1994). Racism can affect health by adversely affecting psychological and physiological functioning and by reducing access to desirable health-enhancing resources such as good housing and medical services. Krieger (1990) has found that the stress of experiencing racial discrimination is positively related to hypertension among African American women, and two studies of Hispanic women have also documented that racial discrimination is a common experience that has pervasive effects on their mental health functioning (Amaro, Russo, & Johnson, 1987; Salgado de Snyder, 1987). The conceptual development of appropriate measures of racism and the empirical assessment of its relationship to health are important issues for enhancing our understanding of the health status of women of color. Meleis and Hattar-Pollara (Chapter 9, this volume) have also reminded us that politicism is a related construct that can significantly affect the health of immigrant women of color.

Research that will advance our knowledge of the health status of various groups of women of color must seek to identify the ways in which socioeconomic position, cultural factors, and racism shape the living conditions and life experiences of women and give rise to particular coping patterns and health outcomes.

Policy Implications

The research reviewed also outlines an important policy agenda for future research on the health of women of color. As Giachello (Chapter 2, this volume) persuasively argues, effectively addressing the health care needs of women of color will require changes in policies, practices, and organizations. Women of color must be more actively involved at every level in shaping health care policy, delivery, and research. This greater involvement on the part of women of color includes planning and directing community-level interventions, serving on advisory boards, holding decision-making positions in organizations, and creating more opportunities for the development of health care providers and support staff from indigenous communities.

The need for culturally sensitive and competent research was another important theme in the earlier chapters of this volume. Appropriately, it has been emphasized that cultural sensitivity applies not only to the delivery of health care and the need for more culturally relevant research but also to the involvement of subjects as full partners in research. However, women must be included in medical research not only as subjects but also as leaders. Several authors indicate that including women of color in positions of power is necessary to reshape the health agenda. History teaches us that the research questions that get asked and the projects that get funded are importantly determined by the social and cultural biases of those who sit in decision-making positions. For example, it is very likely that Dr. Marion Sims, who pioneered techniques of gynecological surgery by keeping a cadre of Negro slaves for the sole purpose of surgical experimentation, would not have gotten his research off the ground if it had been reviewed by a panel of black women. Thus, the inclusion of women of color in decision-making positions in the research infrastructure can change the nature, scope, and emphasis of current research. At the same time, it must be recognized that such inclusion requires the redistribution of power; as the current debates around affirmative action reveal, such proposals are likely to encounter considerable resistance.

Whether the focus is on racial or ethnic populations, women in prison, or homeless women, a golden thread running through this volume is the need for a greater emphasis on prevention in the research and medical treatment of women. A recent analysis of the ambulatory care systems in 10 industrialized nations rated the primary care system of the United States lower than that of all the other countries (Starfield, 1991). Thus, there is a general problem with the delivery of primary care services in the United States that is further compounded for women of color because of their greater health needs.

A health care system that provides comprehensive and coordinated care for women of color requires increased attention to the development and recruitment of primary care physicians. In the last 30 years, there has been a dramatic decline in the production of primary care physicians in the United States, which now has the lowest ratio of primary care physicians to subspecialists of any country in the developed world (Moore, 1991). In Canada, for example, there are 11 primary care physicians for every 10,000 people, compared to 6 in the United States; 68% of all practicing physicians in Canada are in primary care, compared to 35% in the United States (Smith & Anderson, 1990). In England, half of all physicians specialize in primary care, and they provide more than 80% of all ambulatory care contacts, for less than 20% of that country's total health care bill (Moore, 1991).

Health insurance plans also need to be changed to place greater emphasis on disease prevention. Most current insurance policies do not provide reimbursement for many preventive health services. A combination of no insurance or underinsurance and inadequate economic resources, as well as the settings in which health care is disproportionately received, ensure that many under-served women of color receive few preventive services. They are at greatest risk for poor health outcomes and would benefit most from access to preventive primary care.

Several selections in this volume also highlight the neglect of the problem of domestic violence by major social institutions within society. According to some estimates, domestic violence accounts for 20% of all medical visits and 30% of all emergency room visits. Although injuries from domestic violence follow an identifiable pattern, studies show that only 1 in every 25 battered women entering a hospital emergency room is identified as having been a victim of domestic violence. These data highlight the urgent need for routine victimization screening on the part of health care professionals. Currently, most health care settings do not do routine screenings for a history of victimization. Many physicians simply itemize injuries and do not inquire about the context in which these injuries were received or about the possibility that there is an ongoing danger to the patient. Even within the mental health profession, standard procedures for assessment do not include routine questions about physical and sexual abuse.

The contributors to this volume raise fundamental questions about the extent to which all people in our society, irrespective of gender or race or other social characteristics, are accorded equal access to the benefits of our society. They address questions not only about equal access to the desirable resources and rewards in society, but they also outline a broad range of strategies for reducing inequalities in the basic processes and outcomes.

References

Adler, N. E., Boyce, T., Chesney, M. A., Cohen, S., Poldman, S., Kahn, R. L., & Syme, S. L. (1994). Socioeconomic status and health: The challenge of the gradient. *American Psychologist, 49*, 15-24.

Amaro, H., Russo, N. F., & Johnson, J. (1987). Family and work predictors of psychological well-being among Hispanic women professionals. *Psychology of Women Quarterly, 11*, 505-521.

Bunker, J.P., Gomby, D. S., & Kehrer, B. H. (Eds.). (1989). *Pathways to health: The role of social factors.* Menlo Park, CA: Henry J. Kaiser Family Foundation.

Cooper, R. (1984). A note on the biological concept of race and its application in epidemiologic research. *American Health Journal, 108*(3), 715-723.

Cooper, R. S. (1993). Health and the social status of Blacks in the United States. *Annual Epidemiology, 3,* 137-144.

Duster, T. (1984). A social frame for biological knowledge. In T. Duster & K. Garrett (Eds.), *Cultural perspectives on biological knowledge* (pp. 1-40). Norwood, NJ: Ablex.

James, S. A. (1993). Racial and ethnic differences in infant mortality and low birth weight. *Annual Review of Epidemiology, 3,* 130-136.

Krieger, N. (1987). Shades of difference: Theoretical underpinnings of the medical controversy on Black/White differences in the United States, 1830-1870. *International Journal of Health Services, 17,* 259-278.

Krieger, N. (1990). Racial and gender discrimination: Risk factors for high blood pressure? *Social Science Medicine, 30*(12), 1273-1281.

Krieger, N., Rowley, D. L., Herman, A. A., Avery, B., & Phillips, M. T. (1993). Racism, sexism, and social class: Implications for studies of health, disease, and well-being. *American Journal of Preventive Medicine, 9*(supp.), 82-122.

Maxwell, B., & Jacobson, M. (1989). *Marketing disease to Hispanics.* Washington, DC: Center for Science in the Public Interest.

Moore, G. T. (1991). Let's provide primary care to all uninsured Americans—Now! *Journal of the American Medical Association, 265,* 2108-2109.

Salgado de Snyder, V. N. (1987). Factors associated with acculturative stress and depressive symptomatology among married Mexican immigrant women. *Psychology of Women Quarterly, 11,* 475-488.

Scully, D. (1980). *Men who control women's health: The miseducation of obstetricians-gynecologists.* Boston: Houghton Mifflin.

Smith, D. R., & Anderson, R. J. (1990). Community-responsive medicine: A call for a new academic discipline. *Journal of Health Care for the Poor and Underserved, 1,* 219-228.

Starfield, B. (1991). Primary care and health: A cross national comparison. *Journal of the American Medical Association, 266,* 2268.

Vega, W. A., & Amaro, H. (1994). Latino outlook: Good health, uncertain prognosis. *Annual Review of Public Health, 15,* 39-67.

Williams, D. R. (1990). Socioeconomic differentials in health: A review and redirection. *Social Psychology Quarterly, 53*(2), 81-99.

Williams, D. R. (Ed.). (in press). Special issue on racism and health. *Ethnicity and Disease, 5.*

Williams, D. R., & Collins, C. (1995). U.S. socioeconomic and racial differences in health: Patterns and explanations. *Annual Review of Sociology, 21,* 349-386.

Williams, D. R., Lavizzo-Mourey, R., & Warren, R. C. (1994). The concept of race and health status in America. *Public Health Reports, 109*(1), 26-41.

Appendix
Women of Color in the 104th U.S. Congress

African American

HOUSE (10)

Corrinne Brown (D-FL)
Eva Clayton (D-NC)
Barbara Rose Collins (D-MI)
Cardiss Collins (D-IL)
Eddie Bernice Johnson (D-TX)
Sheila Jackson Lee (D-TX)
Cynthia McKinney (D-GA)
Carrie Meek (D-FL)
Eleanor Holmes Norton (D-DC)
Maxine Waters (D-CA)

SENATE (1)

Carol Moseley-Braun (D-IL)

Latina

HOUSE (3)

Ileana Ros-Lehtinen (D-FL)
Lucille Roybal-Allard (D-CA)
Nydia Velazquez (D-NY)

Asian and Pacific Islander

HOUSE (1)

Patsy Mink (D-HI)

Total Women of Color: 15

Author Index

Subject Index

Abused women. *See* Battered women
Accidents:
    as cause of death among African
      American, 123
    as cause of death among Chinese
      American, 73
    as cause of death among Pacific
      Islanders, 73
Acculturation:
    alcohol consumption and, 47
    and behavioral risk factors for
      Hispanics/Latinos, 46-48
    and knowledge of health status of
      women of color, 243
    and psychosocial stressors among
      Asian/Pacific Island women, 102-105
    and substance abuse by
      Asian/Pacific Islanders, 98
    as multidimensional process, 243
    linear, 48
ACT-UP (AIDS activist group), 12
Affirmative action, 5, 9
    and African Americans, 116

definition of, 8
African American households,
    female-headed, 190
African American neighborhoods,
    poverty in, 190
African American population growth, 10
African Americans, 9
    accidental deaths in, 123
    anxiety in, 191
    cancer deaths in, 113, 116, 123
    cancer in, 123
    cardiovascular disease deaths in, 123
    causes of death among, 123-128
    cerebrovascular disease in, 123-124
    cirrhosis deaths in, 123
    depression in, 191
    diabetes deaths in, 123
    diabetes mellitus in, 113, 123, 125-126
    hazardous living environments of,
    114
    hazardous work environments of,
    114

About the Editor

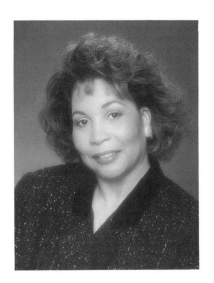

Diane L. Adams, MD, MPH, is Associate Professor in the Department of Physical Therapy at the University of Maryland Eastern Shore, where she teaches Clinical Medicine I. Her areas of specialty include family practice, general preventive medicine, maternal and child health, occupational and environmental health, and public health administration. She is a member of the Johns Hopkins Delta Omega Honorary Society in Public Health—Alpha Chapter, American College of Preventive Medicine, and Alpha Kappa Alpha Sorority, Inc. Dr. Adams is listed in the National Black Health Leadership Directory as one of the top 500 black health professionals in the United States. She serves on numerous professional boards and advisory committees, including the National Consortium for African American Children, Inc. (a former initiative of the National Commission to Prevent Infant Mortality), National Register of Health Service Providers in Psychology, Fielding Institute, and the Urban Health Report. She also serves as the expert medical consultant to Cable 17 Television, Baltimore, Maryland. She served as the first physician Congressional Fellow in the office of Congressman Louis Stokes, as the Chief Medical Officer at the Bureau of Engraving and Printing, and at St. Elizabeths Hospital in Washington, D.C.

Dr. Adams has trained minority health professionals in health policy, legislation and grantsmanship in and outside of the academic setting. She has created several innovative occupational and environmental health programs and minority research centers that have been implemented throughout the public and private sectors. Her research and scholarly activities have focused on health services outcomes research, multicultaralism, cultural diversity, rural, and women's health issues. Her most recent publication, "Living in a Healthy Environment," appears as a chapter in *The Complete Women's Healthbook* (1995). She has an interest in nurturing youth who have the potential to be leaders in our society.

About the Contributors

Linda Burhansstipanov, MSPH, DrPH, CHES, is Director of the Native American Cancer Research Consortium of the American Indian Clinic in Bellflower, California and the Native American Cancer Research Program of the AMC Cancer Research Center in Denver, Colorado. She is the principal investigator of a 3½-year project (1994-1998), "Native American Wellness through Awareness." She is the former director of the Native American Cancer Research Program at the National Institutes of Health. She is a member of several national advisory boards, including the Office of Research for Women's Health, Susan G. Komen Medical Advisory Board and the National Action Plan on Breast Cancer. She is the author of four books, several curricula and numerous articles, and has been actively involved in the women's wellness movement and in Native American health concerns.

Phyllis Old Dog Cross, RN, MS, CARN, is an enrolled member of the Three Affiliated Tribes of Ft. Berthold Reservation in North Dakota. Her tribal affiliation is Mandan-Hidatsa. She has received many awards for her work with Native Americans and women. Most notable were the Wonder Woman Foundation Award and the Gold

Achievement Award from the American Psychiatric Association. She has consulted and published in the areas of transcultural nursing, the health needs of women of color, and the mental health needs of Native Americans and also has consulted as a mental health nurse in the Indian Health Service. She has served on many national boards (as a chartered member of several), including INMED at the University of North Dakota, which recruits and helps Native Americans enter health professions. She has also served as Director of Indian Programs in Futures for Children. She has played a significant role in initiating programs for Native Americans in the areas of suicidal prevention, substance abuse and domestic violence. At present, she is doing volunteer work on her reservation.

Niki Dickerson is a graduate student in sociology at the University of Michigan, Ann Arbor. She has done research on minority health and conducted surveys for public health departments in Texas and Michigan. She has also organized health initiatives in communities of people of color.

Britt K. Ellis, PhD, is Assistant Professor at California State University, Long Beach, where she also is Codirector of the Latino Health Professionals Project in the Health Care Administration Program. She is currently conducting comparative research among Latina immigrant subpopulations concerning infant feeding and care practices. She previously worked in the Department of Health Education at the University of Maryland, College Park, where she taught courses on HIV/AIDS prevention and education and on women's health and nutrition. She has also done research on the HIV/AIDS-related experiences of migrant Latina adolescents.

Patricia Eng, MA, CSW, is a founder and Managing Director of the New York Asian Women's Center, the first organization on the East Coast to comprehensively address domestic violence against Asian American women. The Center offers a 24-hour Asian-multilingual hotline, shelter, counseling, advocacy, and community education programs to a largely immigrant population. As a result of its pioneering efforts, the Center has earned national recognition for its work in the Asian community. Ms. Eng has recieved such prestigious awards as the Susan B. Anthony Award (NOW, NYC), The Gloria Steinem Woman of Vision Award, and the Educational Equity Concepts Groundbreaker Award.

Aida Giachello, MS, PhD, is Associate Professor at the Jane Addams College of Social Work and Director of the Midwest Latino Health, Research, Training, and Policy Center Program (MEDTEP) at the University of Illinois—Chicago. She is an educator, writer, and expert on Hispanic/Latino health care issues. Most of her professional work and research centers on issues of access to medical care, maternal and child health, HIV/AIDS, geriatrics, multicultural issues in health care, and women's health and social issues. Through MEDTEP, she is initiating studies of asthma, diabetes, and pregnancy outcomes. She served as a Special Assistant to the Health Commissioner for Hispanic Affairs for the Chicago Department of Health and served on the National Advisory Committee on Bone Marrow Transplants. She has published extensively both in health policy journals and in newspapers and national magazines.

Marianne Hattar-Pollara, RN, MS, DNSc, is Lecturer at the University of California, Los Angeles, School of Nursing and at California State University, Dominquez Hills. She also serves as consultant to the International Health Program. A native of Amman, Jordan, she helped establish a community-based health service for the Middle Eastern ethnic minority population in the San Francisco Bay area and was involved in developing and coordinating research and clinical training programs for interna

Christine Jose-Kampfner, MS, PhD, is Assistant Professor of Psychology and Education at Eastern Michigan University in Ypsilanti. She is currently conducting research on the special educational needs of Latino youth in urban environments. She has implemented a number of innovative programs for these youth, such as one that brings college students from Eastern Michigan University to Detroit to tutor junior high school students. She has conducted studies on the effects of maternal incarceration and the effects of posttraumatic stress disorder (PTSD) on children who encounter violence. She has published articles and chapters of books on this topic as well as on other issues relating to education in the Latino community. She is cofounder and an active member of the Children's Visitation Program at all women's prisons in the State of Michigan.

Brenda A. Leath, MS, is founding director and Chief Executive Officer of the National Consortium for African American Children (NCAAC), Inc. The Consortium is a multidisciplinary network of national and state organizations working to improve the quality of life for African American children and their families. She also directs the University of the District of Columbia's Family Life Center. She previously had over 12 years of experience in health services administration and has served as Associate Director for Special Population Initiatives at the National Commission to Prevent Infant Mortality; Health Services Administrator Consultant at the Human Services Educational and Research Institute; and Hospital Administrator for the Howard University Hospital Division of Family Practice.

Wilhelmina A. Leigh, PhD, is Senior Research Associate at the Joint Center for Political and Economic Studies in Washington, D.C., specializing in policy research in the areas of health and housing. Previously, she was a Principal Analyst at the U.S. Congressional Budget Office. She has also worked for the Bureau of Labor Statistics, the Department of Housing and Urban Development, the Urban Institute, and the National Urban League Research Department. She has taught at Harvard University, Howard University, and the University of Virginia and is currently an Adjunct Professor at Georgetown University. Her most recent publications include *The Housing Status of Black Americans* (1992), and a report, "The Health Status of Women of Color," which appears as a chapter in *The American Woman (1994-1995), Where We Stand: Women and Health.*

Margaret S. Mason, MS, PhC, is Administrator in the Office of Women's Health, Department of Health and Mental Hygiene, in Baltimore, Maryland. She is also an independent consultant in the areas of cultural sensitivity/diversity, teaching non-verbal gender communication evaluation, program monitoring/evaluation, survey development and analysis, and workshop facilitation. She has had experience as an educator in instructional, administrative, and operational settings in the Baltimore City Public Schools, and she mentors high school children who are in foster care. She is chair of the Baltimore chapter of the National Political Congress of Black Women.

Afaf Ibrahim Meleis, MS, MA, PhD, FAAN, is Professor in the Department of Mental Health, Community, and Administrative Nursing in the School of Nursing, and Associate in Nursing, Nursing Services, at the University of California, San Francisco. Her research focuses on theory and knowledge development, immigrant and international health, and role integration and health. She is the author of over 90 articles, numerous chapters, and an award-winning textbook, *Theoretical Nursing: Development and Progress* (1985, 1991). She has extensive international experience as a visiting professor, speaker, and consultant in the Middle East, Scandinavia, Europe, the Pacific Rim, and South America. Her main teaching areas are theoretical nursing, coping and living with transitions, and international health.

Marian Gray Secundy, MSS, PhD, is Professor and Director of the Program in Clinical Ethics at Howard University College of Medicine, Department of Community Health and Family Practice. She is a practicing family therapist, served as a consultant to the Department of Health and Human Services, and was cochair of a work group in Hillary Rodham Clinton's health care task force. Her research interests include ethical dimensions of patient care, socialization of the medical student, literature and medicine, and minority aging. She has completed an anthology and annotated bibliography of materials by African American writers on topics related to health, illness, aging, and loss and grief, and she has developed curriculum materials for undergraduate courses in bioethics, medical humanities, communication skills, and marital and sexual counseling. She is a member of the boards of numerous national and local organizations and advisory committees at the National Institutes of Health.

Lillian Tom-Orme, PhD, RN, is Director of the Tuberculosis Control/ Refugee Health Program at the Utah Department of Health, Salt Lake City. She frequently serves as consultant to government agencies, including the Division of Nursing, the Office of Minority Health, the

Centers for Disease Control, the Indian Health Service, and several of the National Institutes of Health. A Navajo, she is a highly sought-after speaker on health issues concerning culturally diverse populations, public health, transcultural nursing, tuberculosis, diabetes, and women's health. She has conducted research on the sociocultural aspects of diabetes and breast/cervical cancer in Native American populations. She serves on several national and local boards and advisory councils, including the Board of Directors of the National American Diabetes Association, the Board of Trustees of the Salt Lake Valley Hospitals, the Utah Refugee Advisory Council, and the Advisory Council to Eliminate Tuberculosis.

Reiko Homma True, MSW, PhD, is Assistant Professor of Psychiatry at the University of California, San Francisco. She has played a key role in the development of culturally responsive mental health and substance abuse treatment services for Asian and Pacific Americans in California and in the San Francisco Bay area. She previously served as Deputy Director of Public Health with the San Francisco Department of Public Health; Mental Health Consultant with the National Institute of Mental Health, Region IX; and Director of Adult Services. She directed an Robert W. Johnson Child Health Initiative grant project targeted for immigrant/refugee children and their families, a Department of Health initiative to integrate health, mental health, and substance abuse services. She has an extensive background in pioneering minority health and mental health service development, as well as in the training and teaching of minority and women's concerns in health and clinical psychology.

Shanell Semien is a senior psychobiology major at the University of California at Los Angeles School of Medicine, where she is a member of the Pre-Medical Scholars Institute. She also is a tutor and supervisor of math tutors in the Academic Advancement Program for underrepresented minority and low-income students. A member of Sigma Gamma Rho Sorority, she plans to become an obstetrician/gynecologist.

Shannon Semien is a senior psychobiology major at the University of California at Los Angeles, where she is a member of the Pre-

Medical Scholars Institute. She plans to attend medical school and to become an obstetrician/gynecologist. She is a member of Sigma Gamma Rho Sorority and is a volunteer at Martin Luther King Jr./ Drew Hospital. She is the twin sister of Shanell Semien.

Grace M. Wang, MD, is Assistant Clinical Professor of Family Practice in Pediatrics at the Columbia University College of Physicians and Surgeons and is Medical Director of the Chinatown Health Clinic in New York City. She worked as Medical Director in Family Care Group Practice and the Health Center for Women and Children at St. Luke's\Roosevelt Hospital Center in New York, and as physician at the East Third Street Family Shelter and at the Family Care Center in the Bronx, New York. She has made numerous presentations related to community-oriented primary care for high-risk populations. She is a member of the American Academy of Family Physicians and Clinical Directors Network of Region II.

Betty Smith Williams, DrPH, RN, FAAN, is Professor in the Department of Nursing, California State University, Long Beach. A fellow of the American Academy of Nursing, she is former Dean and Professor in the School of Nursing, University of Colorado Health Science Center. Previously, she was Assistant Dean and Professor in the School of Nursing, University of California, Los Angeles (UCLA). In 1956, she was Professor of Public Health Nursing at Mount St. Mary's College in Los Angeles, where she was the first African American nurse to teach in a California nursing higher degree program. In 1968, she cofounded the Council of Black Nurses in Los Angeles and served as its president for 5 years. She is a founder and charter member of the National Black Nurses Association (NBNA), where she currently serves as parliamentarian and chair of the Health Services Research and chair of the Health·Policy Committee. She is Associate Editor of the Journal of the National Black Nurses Association. In 1985, she was the first African American elected to the Board of Directors of Blue Cross of California. Previously, in 1975, she was the first woman and African American to serve as a Blue Cross of Southern California Director. She is former National Treasurer of Delta Sigma Theta Sorority, Inc. and former president of Delta Sigma Theta Telecommunications, Inc. The NAACP Legal Defense and

Education Fund recognized her in 1991 as a Black Woman of Achievement, and in 1994 she received the Achievement Award of the NBNA for her "vision in the formation of NBNA and continuous mentoring of Black Nurses."

David R. Williams, PhD, MPH, is Associate Professor of Sociology, and an Associate Scientist, Institute for Social Research, the University of Michigan. His previous academic appointment was at Yale University. His research has focused on socioeconomic status differences in health in general, and the health of African American population in particular. He has served as a consultant to numerous federal health agencies and private organizations. Currently he is an Associate Editor of *Ethnicity and Disease*, a member of the National Committee on Vital and Health Statistics and chair of its subcommittee on Minority and Other Special Populations. He is also a member of a National Academy of Sciences and the National Science Foundation's Board of Overseers for the General Social Survey.

Ruth E. Zambrana, PhD, is Enochs Chair Professor and Director of the Center for Child Welfare at George Mason University, College of Nursing and Health Science, in Fairfax, Virginia. She has conducted research for the past 15 years on the health of low-income Latino/Hispanic women, children, and families, with a special focus on maternal and child health. She has published extensively on issues related to health, education, employment, and research methodology among low-income women of color. Her most recent edited book is *Understanding Latino Families: Scholarship, Policy, and Practice* (1995).

About the Artist

Adrian Wong Shue was born in 1952 on the West Indies island of Jamaica. Rich and diverse in the culture of both primitive art brought in from West Africans and the European influence from the early British colonization of Jamaica, Wong Shue explored different approaches to art at an early age. In his preteens, he enjoyed the freedom of painting with mud and smearing flower petals on paper. When he was 14, he studied with Alfred Chin of Canton, China, and developed the love and respect for nature that is so important in Oriental culture. He also acquired an affinity for charcoal drawing. In 1967, he began studying privately with Alexander Cooper, Professor of Art at Kingston College in Jamaica.

Wong Shue's approach to subject matter and his use of materials reflects his dedication to the idea of nonexclusivity. This openminded approach and the free expression it fosters have led the artist to develop a number of painting styles and to use a variety of media, including woodcuts, lino cuts, ink drawing, charcoal, gouache, and oil painting. Using thick Japanese natsume fabric paper allows him to develop textures and patterns in the form of mixed media. The movement over this wet textured paper allows the artist to produce effects difficult to achieve by painting on canvas or board. Wong Shue is best described as in a constant experimental stage. He travels throughout the world and is drawn to local artists and their art forms. He continues to explore mythology, through which he seeks harmony with the universe.

After several trips to Brazil, Wong Shue became concerned for the vanishing culture of the world's rain forests. In 1990, he created *Songs of the Earth*, a series of benefit exhibitions to support the UskoAyar Amazonian school of painting, a free art workshop for the youth of the Amazon. *Songs of the Forest* depicts the modernday martyr, Chico Mendez, who was murdered in Brazil because of his pioneering efforts to stop the attacks on the Brazilian people and the destruction of rain forests. Wong Shue sponsors *Rain Forest Visions*, a touring museum exhibition of UskoAyar art. He is proud to support efforts to establish "eco-sustainability." Wong Shue's work has been exhibited throughout the United States and internationally. He continues to paint both from his Los Angeles studio and from around the world.